It's Not About The Whip

Love, Sex, and Spirituality in the BDSM Scene

By Sensuous Sadie

SensuousSadie@aol.com
www.sensuoussadie.com

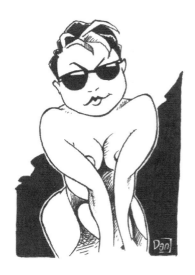

© Copyright 2003 Sensuous Sadie. All rights reserved.

No part of this book may be reproduced, stored in a retrieval system, or transmitted, in any form or by any means, electronic, mechanical, photocopying, recording, or otherwise, without the prior written permission of the author, except for the inclusion of brief quotations in a review.

Cover and Book Design by Sensuous Sadie.

This book is protected under International and Pan-American Copyright Conventions.

```
National Library of Canada Cataloguing in Publication Data

Sensuous Sadie
      It's not about the whip : my explorations into love,
sex and spirituality in the BDSM scene / Sensuous Sadie.
ISBN 1-4120-0183-8
      I. Title.
HQ79.S34 2003      306.77'5'092      C2003-901946-2
```

Published in the United States of America by
Bitch Kitty Books,
in association with

TRAFFORD

This book was published *on-demand* in cooperation with Trafford Publishing. On-demand publishing is a unique process and service of making a book available for retail sale to the public taking advantage of on-demand manufacturing and Internet marketing. **On-demand publishing** includes promotions, retail sales, manufacturing, order fulfilment, accounting and collecting royalties on behalf of the author.

Suite 6E, 2333 Government St., Victoria, B.C. V8T 4P4, CANADA
Phone   250-383-6864   Toll-free   1-888-232-4444 (Canada & US)
Fax   250-383-6804   E-mail   sales@trafford.com
Web site www.trafford.com TRAFFORD PUBLISHING IS A DIVISION OF TRAFFORD
HOLDINGS LTD.
Trafford Catalogue #03-0551   www.trafford.com/robots/03-0551.html

10   9   8   7   6   5   4   3   2

Comments on Sadie's Writing

With her generous spirit and questing intelligence, Sadie isn't satisfied merely to have been there and done that – she needs to find out what it all means. Her insights will help speed many others along on their own journeys toward sexual self-revelation.
~ *Gary Switch, Contributing Editor, Prometheus*

It means a great deal to me to have my writing and activism understood by someone who is going to be continuing this work after I am gone. I also just loved the phrase "think globally, spank locally," and feel that it should probably be a t-shirt and a bumper sticker if not a prime time TV show. What a great way to sum up the ways in which we must build community while seeking out our own pleasure. You're just a peach. Thanks so much for a brilliant and impassioned effort. Once more you have my admiration and best wishes.
~ *Patrick Califia, Author & Activist*

It's very educating to get into Sadie's mind through her writings. She definitely has a unique and refreshing view on what we do.
~ *Sir Victor, Leader of DomSubFriends of New York City*

That is a great column! I think you hit it right on the head. We can't turn away from our sexual activism because of things happening outside our community, and we do need to support our activists who give so much to help create a better world for all of us. You're really doing your part to activate our community.
~ *Susan Wright, Founder of the National Coalition for Sexual Freedom*
[Referring to *Think Globally, Spank Locally*]

Sadie's down-to-earth lifestyle observations will have experienced players nodding their heads, and provide the beginner with an invaluable guide to the multi-faceted world of D/s-BDSM. Her explorations of the spirituality of kink and her willingness to share her personal experiences add substance and sizzle to this collection of essays.
~ *Elizabeth, Board Member of Rose & Thorn of Vermont*

Sensuous Sadie's website not only offers the best collection of writings on the web examining the intersection of the spirit and sadoerotic, but it is also simply one of the most illuminating collections of SM writings period. Think of it as a continuation of the essays of Mark Thompson's "Leatherfolk" tailored to the cyber age and the new millennium. Simply Wonderful!
~ *Chris M, writer and Emeritus Board Member of Black Rose, Washington DC*

It is evident that Sadie's writing comes from the heart of someone in the D/s lifestyle. It's nice for a change to have someone with experience in what they write.
~ *Angel Babee, Leader of Sisters in Submission*

Sadie's scene writings are fresh, witty and observant.
~ *Mayafire, Co-Leader of Albany Power Exchange (APeX), of New York*

Sadie writes with compassion and conviction about the complexities of BDSM. Her writing has given voice to the needs and dreams of our community.
~ *Jonathan, Executive Director of Rose & Thorn of Vermont*

Even though I read Sadie's columns on House Mermaid as they emerged, a strange thing happened when I edited the book for her; I found I could not put the book down. Sadie has the ability to translate her experiences into writing, a rare gift.
~ *Dex, Master of House Mermaid*

Your writing voice is clear without being strident and the breezy tone helps keep the "sturm und drang" out of what is surely a subject filled with a bit too much of that. Most of what I read on the web is so hopelessly cloying, overdone or just plain bad, so this a refreshing counterpoint.
~ *Anne Marie Delaney*

Sadie analyzes the male/female demographics of BDSM and provides the reader with valuable advice as to how to make them work for you.
~ *Ed, Leader of White Mountains Different Strokes of New Hampshire*

Sensuous Sadie is an exceptional writer, with a zest for the lifestyle few have.
~ *Lady Bleu, Editor of DomSubLifestyle Online*

I find Sensuous Sadie's writing style an easy to read and refreshing view of the BDSM lifestyle from a real time player. She is a great resource with her perspective from both the top and the bottom.
~ *Lord Battista, Erotic Power Exchange Dominion*

Sadie is possibly the most vibrant and informed individual on the internet today. She never sleeps due to a surgically implanted device that allows her to labor tirelessly on her newsletter, her website, her very fascinating interviews, her BDSM writers Yahoo group, her leadership of Rose & Thorn, and very likely 30 or 40 more BDSM related activities I haven't yet run across. I respect her for her strong opinions, and for being able to convey them without diminishing the validity of other ideas.
~ *yielding, BDSM Columnist*

Intriguing , Interesting, Insightful, Poignant and Enlightening. A thought provoking style that will make you want to read it more then once.
~ *Charlie, Associate Editor of the BDSM News*

It is with the greatest of pleasure that I comment on Sensuous Sadie's work. Having featured her work on the BDSM Resource Center has seen a dynamic increase in positive comments on the fresh views that she shares. Sadie brings her style to the written word and her style is just that, style and delightfully Sadie. If you are some of the fortunate people that have had access to Sensuous Sadie's literary contributions then you will feast in this compilation of her work. If you have not had that opportunity then you are in for a sumptuous treat! Her slant reflects the lifestyle, on both a personal and community level, in a way that gives food for thought as well as makes you smile.
~ *CC, Editor of the BDSM Resource Center*

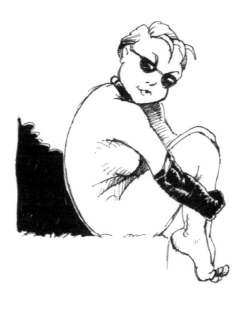

*Look, if you want to torture me,
spank me, lick me, do it.
But if this poetry shit continues
just shoot me now please.*
~ Lori Petty in Tank Girl

Acknowledgements

I'd like to thank my spiritual sister Leela. Together we have explored both the mundane and the transcendent.

Thank you to my professional writing coach K.K. Wilder for her invaluable assistance in bringing this book to press. She's quite the taskmistress, at least in the writing arena.

Thank you Dan Dofogh for the wonderful renderings of Sadie Sez and the chastity cartoon. Please visit Dan's website at www.dandofogh.com.

Thank you to Chris M., author and artist for rendering my design of the snake BDSM logo. More of his art and spirituality writings can be found on his website at http://subbondage.net/chris_m.

I'd like to thank Dex and the family at House Mermaid for generously opening their house and their hearts to me. Dex was also kind enough to give me ongoing feedback on my writing. Readers interested in contacting him can do so through his website www.housemermaid.com.

Thank you to fetish photographers Magnum (front cover), David Southwick (back cover) and Versive (inside photo). All of you have a marvelous ability to make me look totally hot!

I have long enjoyed the support and interest of the Vermont community in my endeavors. Thank you to everyone who have helped make my explorations real.

I love words, and especially appreciate the phrase "Erotica Mystica," courtesy of Neil.

Real and scene names are included according to the wishes of the authors. All other names have been changed.

~ *Sensuous Sadie*

SensuousSadie@aol.com
www.sensuoussadie.com

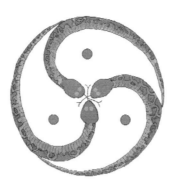

Introduction

I first started exploring Dominance and submission with my friend Bailey. We went camping one summer in the White Mountains of New Hampshire, and in the dark of the tent we shared our secret fantasies. I told him about wanting to be controlled in a sexual manner, although I didn't really know what that meant. Bailey knew. To my extreme embarrassment he ordered me to masturbate, right there in the tent, right there in front of him. Then, when I was just short of orgasm, he made me stop. When I had cooled down, he started all over again. This feeling of being so close and then not being allowed release created an erotic pain, a submission that thrilled me. I wanted more.

This would be the experience that turned me on to the world of BDSM: Bondage & Discipline; Dominance & Submission; and Sadism & Masochism

When Bailey and I started looking for information on what we were doing, we found the book *Screw the Roses, Send me the Thorns*, which is still my favorite, not only for its content, but also for its lighthearted approach. Today there are many books on safety, apparatus, and erotica, but few that explore the power exchange from an emotional and spiritual point of view. Yet, it is this transformational aspect that makes my heart and body sing.

As I explored this lifestyle, I began to see how my BDSM experiences had a relationship to my spiritual path. I would describe my spiritual approach as Taoist in nature, with a relativist twist. This is why I capitalize both Dominant and Submissive; because just as in the yin/yang symbol, they are equal and interlocked parts of each other. Going into subspace isn't just kinky sex for me, although it sure does turn me on. It's also an entre into a mystical place similar to a walking meditation. The everyday world recedes, and I become more in touch with my own nature and with my higher power. Through exploring my BDSM orientation, I became more grounded and focused.

This book is a collection of columns that I wrote over the last few years as I recovered from a very painful breakup (just like a country song). The first section includes my personal reflections about being a Submissive, a Switch, and yes, a Dominant too. The second section includes the writing I've done in some unconventional, and sometimes controversial areas. The third section, Dating in the Scene follows the somewhat entertaining stories of my dating life. The fourth section, Diary of a Journalist Submissive, is the story about my experience at House Mermaid. In the fifth section I write about how the BDSM community has changed my views about our place in society. Finally, I write about being "Sensuous Sadie," and how being a leader and a writer has changed my life.

I'm hoping my travels through these strange and mystical places will light your path as well.

~ *Sensuous Sadie*

Table Of Contents:

Part I - My Submissive Nature
It's Not About the Whip – Exploring the Erotica
Mystica of BDSM 2
My Submissive Nature 7
Thanksgiving Submission 11
Getting Slapped 14
Considering a 24/7 Relationship 16
Just Call Me a Bedroom Submissive 23
Between Domspace and Subspace 26
Vicarious Submission 29

Part II: Unconventional Explorations
Born a Hoochie Mama and Where I Got those Crazy
Ideas 34
Fat Women, Body Image, and Sexual Politics in the
BDSM Scene 39
The Nature of Sadism and the Sadism of my Nature 45
Meeting the Devil at the Crossroads of Spirituality,
Sexuality, Love, and BDSM 49
Adultery, Betrayal, and How I Rationalized My Way
Out Of Things 53
Strong Female Submissives 56
The Submissive in Charge 60
Submissives who Train their Dominants 65
Steamy True Stories of Dominating and Submitting
(with a little poetic license) 69

Part III: Dating in the Scene
The Single Submissive's Lament 74
Novice on the Precipice 78
Can a Kinky Girl Date A Straight Guy? The Story of my
Vacation in Vanillaland 82
Going on a Dating Sabbatical, and the One Who Slipped
in Under the Wire 86

Part IV: Diary of a Journalist Submissive: My Adventures in Formal BDSM Training

Exploring the Possibility of Formal Training 90
Why This? 93
The First Weekend 96
Dex and Me 100
My PolySomething Relationships 105
Cupid, Collars, and Commitment 111
Morphing into the Group .115
Drunk on Chastity 119
Stepping Out 124
So What Do You Feel about All This? 129
It Ain't Entirely a Bowl of Cherries 133
Closure 137

Part V: Relationships & Community

Think Globally, Spank Locally 142
BDSM Relationships: Vanilla with a Dash of Kink, or a Whole Different Animal? 148
How to Spot a Dominant at Ten Paces 154
Sadie Comes Out as a Bawdy Girl 162
Rough Sex, BDSM, and other Mushy Deliniations .169
Sobriquets and Screen Names:
What we Call Ourselves 172
Making Sense of Internet Writing Styles 177
Why I Don't Give a Hoot about Protocol and Why It's Important to Know Anyway 184

Part VI: Becoming Sensuous Sadie

SCENEprofiles Interview with Sensuous Sadie . . .190
Arrogant, Hysterical, and Nearly Insane: Being a BDSM Writer 207
Top Three Reasons Why Readers Think I'm Full-o-Hooey 211
Controversial, Me? 216

Appendix

Glossary of BDSM Terms .221
About the Author 227
Why I Self Published this Book 229

Part I - My Submissive Nature

Some of my writing is practical, but much of it is about what's happening inside me as I explore different kinds of relationships. To write about an experience as it's happening – not weeks or months later – gives it energy and magic.

Quite a few people have commented on what they call my "courage" for publishing such personal stories. I don't really see it as courage because when you're a writer, it's just plain what you do. But there's something else, too. There's nothing quite as special as knowing you've reached another person, way down deep inside where he or she doesn't often venture. That's the part of writing which keeps me going.

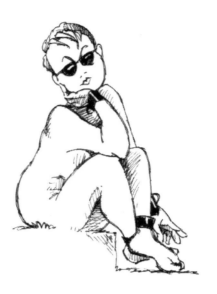

It's Not About The Whip - Exploring The Erotica Mystica Of BDSM

Imagination is more important than knowledge
~ Einstein

My first Dominant owned one toy, a leather slapper I bought at a sex shop, a toy that regularly got lost in the murky depths of his car. The thing was, we didn't need any toys, and could not have imagined the wealth of accoutrements now found in my closet. Our D/s experience was the stuff of dreams: exploratory, magical, transformative, scary.

On our first night together, I sat waiting to see if he would take the reins, to take me. He stood behind me, and I smelled the scent of his passion. I felt his breath, his heartbeat. So, too, did I feel his indecision, his own question about how best to proceed. Secretly, I wanted to feel a cool breeze around my ankles, telling me that he'd walked away to watch the rest of the hockey game; to grill up some shish kabobs; to shovel the driveway. I was afraid of this dark realm which yawned ahead. I couldn't quite put my finger on what it was or where I was going. I was lost in a breathless moment of sitting on that fence, not knowing... not knowing. A moment still and silent in my memory, even now.

Then, Bailey lifted my chin so my eyes could meet his. I saw the decision there, clear and intent. Knowing he had decided, I did, too. I relaxed into him.

Bailey and I traveled this D/s path without benefit of paddles, whips, and floggers. We did it with only a bit of information from the just-born Internet. We did it knowing nothing, less than nothing, about etiquette, safety, technique, protocol, or equipment of any sort. Instead, we had common sense, which in the end, turned out to be all we needed.

Today, after years of being a leader of a BDSM group, I have a boxful of toys: floggers and paddles and wax and rope. Condoms and clamps and crops. Spreader bars and scarves. What I do not have at the moment, is a man like Bailey to look into my eyes and tell me I'm his. But if I did, I know he wouldn't be about the "stuff." He too would be a mystic, an explorer on a path of shadows dappled from an overhang of heavy boughs, a path made apparent only by the empty branches of blueberries eaten along the way.

It wasn't just toys I collected along the way. I also learned about BDSM safety and etiquette, enough perhaps to take a step up to more edgy play, enough to prevent making a fool of myself. The demonstrations at our parties are the kind easy to do in public: not much skin, not much intense sexuality, not much overt humiliation. Nevertheless, after a few years, I have the feeling that for so many scene folk, the power exchange has come to be about the apparatus, not about the experience.

Let me be completely clear here; education and safety are important. If you are going to tie someone up, you have to do it right or you risk hurting them. Same with flogging. But techniques and safety knowledge are simply the essential basics, elementary mechanics. That car will run fine, but I want to go to the moon.

It's also true that if you go to a play party, or otherwise join the larger BDSM community, you need to know proper manners and etiquette for each type of event you attend. For these reasons, many BDSM groups see education as their mission. Education is a good thing, but if that's all there is, BDSM becomes form without substance.

In contrast, my approach has been to build a community and provide a safe space to explore our sexual identities. For many of us, D/s is not just about the toys, but rather the emotional and spiritual transformation occurring within, where the mind and soul surrender. My approach is of an artist, more interested in the expression than in who made the paint.

The usual way to get to this place is through the body as vehicle, using tactile sensation and sensual stimulation. It invokes a shift in perception, a shift from the daily world pronounced enough to enter the realm of Dom, or subspace. I wonder about approaching that door not through stimulating the body, but through the silken pathway of the soul. That's the mystica I seek, where he and I meet through the translucent waves of voice, of touch, of scent, of magic.

I don't care about floggers; which way they're made or how much they cost. I want to feel my blood rising to the surface with a tingle, rising to meet another stroke.

I don't care about the fifteen ways to tie a person to the door. I want to feel not the pressure and pull of the rope against my skin, but rather the helplessness slipping between my legs, opening me wide so I am without barriers.

I don't care about whether or not protocol tells me to gaze this way or that, to speak or not, to wear this color flag or another to announce my intentions. I care about hearing his whisper, close from the chattering crowd, close enough to hear his possession of my sexuality, my strength, my self.

What I want to explore is not the "stuff" of BDSM, but the enchantment. The trembling feeling that wakes me far past midnight in a sheen of heat.

But still I am dragged back to the practical. Novices write me for recommendations about what they should buy in the way of BDSM gadgets, and I send them a list; the usual suspects.

What I'd really like to give them is a list of mental, spiritual, and emotional qualities to bring to the table. I'd tell them to bring joy, creativity, and enthusiasm. Bring caring and patience and a commitment to communicating, even when it's a hassle. Bring not what you think a Dominant should be, but rather your own passion to dominate cleanly and without measure. Bring awareness of your self and a willingness to face your own fears. Bring yourself present, genuine and alive and here in this very moment.

Bring your questions.

If you are a Dominant, how will you discover what makes your Submissive's world "go round?" What can you do to create a whole new awareness for your Submissive? How will you care for her or his emotional well being? How will you deal with the vulnerable place they will be in, not only during a scene, but even as early as the first time you meet and feel that little tingle?

How will you learn to read your Submissive's reactions, physical and non-physical so you can teasingly torment them into a state of mindless sensual bliss? How will you learn to play your Submissive's body like a fine violin, to compose a symphony of subspace?

If you are a Submissive, your responsibilities are different; your questions different. How do you protect your inner self enough to negotiate fully with this person, while still opening up enough to let yourself be known? How do you learn to trust being vulnerable when so many Dominants don't have the emotional skills to cope with garden variety emotions, much less the profound ones of D/s play? When will you tell this person about your sexual and BDSM preferences? If you do it too early, you will not have kept to your personal boundaries about privacy and intimacy, but if you hold back too long, your Dominant won't have the necessary information. Are you caring for yourself enough, so your Dominant doesn't have to rescue you? Do you know who you are and what takes you to that magical place so you can communicate this to your partner? What is subspace really about for you?

If our life journeys unfolded in a straight line, we would each have an unambiguous path ahead. But D/s, like life, is a series of parallel paths instead. For me, its transcendent nature begs to be explored, not through apparatus, but through the hush of his breath on my neck, the linger of his hand in my hair, and the soft and steady resonance of his voice leading me to our destination.

My Submissive Nature

People often tell me stories about when they first realized they were Submissive or Dominant. In my own case there wasn't a particular instant when I recognized my own orientation, but rather it grew from unassuming moments, the kind that I'd dredge up fifteen years later for opening gambits to my stories. But I do remember when I fell off the fence and crossed over permanently from vanilla to D/s.

For many years I was mildly bored with vanilla sex. While my lovers were invariably imaginative, I was irritated and impatient with the loving "slow hand" of foreplay. My tastes have always run to the rough and tumble, but it's more than that, much more. They wanted to please me, but secretly I wanted to be forced to please them. They wanted me to have multiple orgasms; I wanted my sexuality to be controlled, limited. They wanted to caress; I wanted to be spanked until I wept.

One day I met and seduced Chris, mostly because he looked how I imagined a Dominant would look. Tall and muscular, he sported black muscle shirts and a James Dean air. He had been in jail for some obscure offense, a bad boy who appealed to the suburban Jersey girl in me. One day, a few months into the affair, I observed him hanging some plants off the porch roof. I suggested in a playful way that rather than hanging plants, he tie me to those plant hooks and have his way with me. His response was that he could never tie me up, much less do more; it simply wasn't in his nature. No matter how much I tried to convince him the act would be consensual, he refused.

That night, I had a long talk with myself. I liked this man, maybe even loved him, but I knew I could not make a commitment to a person who could never satisfy me sexually.

I wanted more than I was getting, and it was time to start dating only men who were in alignment with my needs. I made a commitment to myself and sealed it with a silver ring, which I wore on my ring finger. It was a silver lion's head with garnet eyes sparkling with mischief. Like all decisions, it opened up new paths of exploration. I could not have imagined how this commitment, this ring would affect my life, from starting a BDSM community to writing a book on my experiences.

Of course in the beginning, I didn't have a clear idea about what exactly I wanted or how to get it. Most of the men I dated were what some people call "vanilla Dominants," regular Joes with a commanding streak. Usually this translated into a little silk scarf bondage and a slap on the fanny. Never enough, not for me. Like most novices, I sampled flavors with a tiny pink spoon and picked a few favorites.

I also began to spend more time thinking about my nature and how it fits into the scheme of things. For some players, sex is not part of the D/s equation, or maybe a minor part. For me, sex is the foundation of the submissive experience. In short, submitting turns me on. My submissive nature is a sexual orientation, much as being lesbian or gay. I also observed that the Dominants I knew either had it or they didn't. I came to the conclusion that this orientation is hard wired in, and because of this awareness I would never again try to convert a vanilla partner to the lifestyle. These choices have limited me in some ways and also freed me. As I have turned myself over to my nature, I have become more directed as a person. More confident, more expressive, more myself. It's the same as when I turn myself over to the spirit within me. Because I know I am in safe hands, I am able to make choices free of fear. At first, I thought that making a commitment to a particular path would rule out other options, limiting me. In fact, committing to something allowed me to go much farther and deeper on my own path, my right path. It's not that there are less choices available, rather that I have focused myself on where I am going. On both the spiritual and sexual levels, I see the path before me and am following it faithfully. Subspace is not a destination, but a process of exploring my spiritual way.

There have been a few times when I visited a magical place, more magical than subspace. There was no stumbling or hesitation, but rather like the "zipless fuck" where one's clothes fall off effortlessly. I'm not sure what exactly made these moments happen, whether it was the Dominant's style or something opening up in me, or maybe a confluence of both. All the elements were in place: his experience level, his confidence, and his knowing exactly what needed to be done. My readiness.

Some people might call me a lifestyler, but I don't really see myself that way. While I'm more involved in the lifestyle than most, the practice of BDSM is not the larger part of who I am. For a long time I saw my orientation as a hobby, something I did on the side. It's more now, if only because I spend so much time thinking and writing about it, but it's not the balance of my life, only the balance of my writing at the moment. My writing is more about self-exploration than it is about BDSM, even when I'm writing about BDSM.

Through this process of sorting things out and writing about them, I found out how to articulate what I believe about my own submissive nature. I believe that submitting is a solitary act, something to be shared only with my Dominant. Playing in public turns my gift into theatre.
 Submitting is a sacred quest, not something to be shared with just anyone who asks. I will give myself only to someone who shares my path. Serving is a spiritual expression which lifts me above the mundane. I will put aside my own needs to serve his. When I can be vulnerable, it is the deepest expression of my submission, and of myself. When I can trust my partner completely: physically, emotionally, and spiritually, then my soul can take flight.
 There may not be a moment when everything comes into focus. There have been a hundred moments which inch-wormed me one bit closer to understanding my nature, my self. I get it now, and only have to wait patiently for Him to find me.

Submission on Thanksgiving Night

One of my mother's favorite stories was about her dating days. On the way to a snowy dinner date she and her gentleman-friend, as she called him, stopped at his place to pick up a warmer coat. When he returned from the other room he was buck naked. With nary a raised eyebrow, my mother thanked him nicely and left the house. The moral of the story is that men were horndogs and I shouldn't be surprised by some pretty offbeat behavior. What I actually learned was that a lady leaves when it's time, and never forgets to say thank you.

So I wasn't all that surprised when the same thing happened to me. I was at my friend Diego's house prior to a Thanksgiving dinner out. He mentioned that he was running late and ran upstairs to take a quick shower. He also asked me to pick out a snazzy outfit for him from his neatly organized closet (yes, he's submissive). I chose a brown and blue tweed jacket with a pair of tightly-fitted black pants. I call these kind of trousers "gay" pants because they'd surely attract attention from the gay boys, not that that would bother Diego any (yes, he's bisexual). As I was rustling through the belts, Diego finished his shower and out he came, stark naked!

As I stared at him, my mother's dating story popped into my mind, not the slightest bit faded for twenty years in between tellings. Was I lady enough to thank Diego nicely and leave the house? This had never happened to me before, so I said a little prayer to my mother in heaven, and didn't blink an eye. Instead, I took a gander at Diego's muscular shoulders, firm ass, and remarkably large balls. It was a nice vision, and I figured heck, why not check out the goods before purchase?

After an eyeful, I decided not to walk out, and said instead, "That's one hell of a set of balls you have there, Diego." He grinned at me. No, I wasn't offended, I wanted to throw him to the floor and take him hard. Still, there were those dinner reservations, and mashed potatoes were whispering my name. So I called on the Gods of restraint and turned my attention to choosing a matching pair of shoes.

Diego may or may not have been hitting on me with the nude parade, but as far as I was concerned, sex was already a foregone conclusion. The nice thing about Diego is that he and I are sexual equals, pulsing with a matched energy of the sexual divine. It's not about being horny all the time, but having taken my sexual soul in and made it mine. It's about looking at life through the rosy red lens of sexuality. I don't find this very often, and it's frankly more important than any part of his body, no matter how attractive. A lot of women, including my mother, would have walked out, but Diego and I are matched opponents.

Of course that doesn't stop us from bickering about who's going to be Dominant, being as we are both switches. I think we might be settling on me as Mistress though, which generally works because I like having things my way. Even so, he has the balls, the big balls, to let me know when I've screwed up. I may get peevish, but I listen anyway; because not many people ever tell me to straighten up and fly right. That's a fine quality in a friend, be he Dominant or a Submissive.

You might have thought that after all that, we'd have returned home to fuck until the ropes frayed. Instead, we spent the dark wee hours of Thanksgiving cuddling. Although we seemed to have settled on him dominating that evening, one of the more memorable moments came when I was on top, gazing down with lust in my heart, him looking up with that exquisitely tender expression that only a Submissive can have. As I kissed him, I felt him soar free into the night, just a moment or two before coming back. His eyes were soft and dark, and I wanted to hold him close, closer. I wanted to cradle him in my hands like a water lily, vulnerable and open, sparkling with dew. I wanted to lick the dew off, savor the sweetness, press its cool petals against my cheek.

No, it wasn't the buck-naked body that got me, it was that look, silent and aching.

I think my mom would be proud of me. Not of how I handled a streaker before dinner, but how I can stay present when something magical is happening right in front of me. Later on when it was time, I left, and yes, I thanked him.

Getting Slapped

One evening a few years ago my Master slapped me. It wasn't all that hard a slap, but it was in the face and I was so shocked, I just couldn't think for a moment. Then there was a little switch which flipped over, and I sank into subspace with a little murmur.

I suppose if I had thought about face slapping before, I would have said it was out of the question. I would have said I'd slap back. But I didn't. I didn't because at the moment it happened, on my knees in front of him, I was freed from my self and invited into the mysterious.

The intense joy of submitting your self to another is hard to describe. In turning over the power, I and Thou disappear and we merge into something more powerful, more vibrant than either of us alone. I yearn for he who can lead me there, take me to the next level. Not another Dominant wannabe who can't control his own life, much less mine, but a man with power and imagination and confidence.

The beauty in belonging to someone, knowing they are your protector and leader, is a confidence of an unusual flavor. It's not dependence, the kind which sometimes gets us into trouble, but rather an interdependence which strengthens us both.

On the surface it might look like passiveness, but true submission is a conscious, assertive act. He works with me to help me grow. He recognizes my gift to him. He sees my whole, true self.

In exchange I give what I can in service, in pleasure, and in pain. I wait on him physically and in other ways. I anticipate his needs and fill them. I serve his pleasure without wanting anything for myself. In releasing my own wants, I am freed.

I eagerly accept his control of my pleasure. He allows me pleasure only when I have proven myself and served well, but often not even then because it puts the focus on me instead of him. While pain is simply endured, a withdrawal of pleasure is deeper and more ephemeral, a hard thing to measure. It follows me in the times when submitting is not what's on my mind; in my office, at the grocery store or at a dinner party. By turning over my childish need for instant gratification, I grow spiritually.

He also believes in regular punishment because it keeps the demarcation straight; it keeps me in line. There are few things in this life so clearly delineated and so clearly appreciated for the gift they are. When I experience pain for him, it is transformed into pleasure. With each crack of a paddle or a crop, another small piece of my own insisting demanding self is released.

At the moment he slapped me, all these things came into play. That's why I didn't slap back. That's why.

Considering a 24/7 Relationship

I feel a vibration trilling up from my soul. It is a humming, soft and dark. My nerves are on edge, my head swims. It is not lust or love, I know those things well enough to know they are not this. It is deeper, elemental, and primal. I am powerful and powerless, my blood pulsing through me like a heavy rainstorm.

This feeling with no name is the state of true submission for me, and I have felt it only a few times in my life. Along the way of two Dominants, two Submissives and a bunch of one-night-spank-stands, I have savored its flavors from milquetoast to magic. It is a black-tie taste, acquired through grace and a sky of very bright stars.

This week I have asked Tyler to help me experience it 24/7. We discussed doing it for a limited time, a three-week contract which could be renewed so neither of us would feel pressured. This time I want it for more than just a few minutes on a convenient play evening. I want to know what it feels like to have my sexuality controlled, not in a temporary fashion forgotten an hour later, but in a very real, very visceral way. I want to know what it's like to serve someone, not just sexually, but in all ways; not just for the evening, but for the week. I want to know what it's like to really turn it over, not just for fun, but for real.

I want to know what it's like to serve someone of such high caliber. I want him to take me to all the subspace places I've never been. Can he do it? I know he can, at least on the practical level. Does he also have the skills for the emotional wraparound which comes along? I don't know, and maybe he doesn't either. But if he makes that leap, the result will be a powerful dynamic of our interlocking energy.

This is the story of my first 24/7 relationship. But, as negotiations go forward, I've realized my 24/7 desires might not be fulfilled, at least with this person. I'd thought to write about it after the fact, but then it might not even happen. It is common for D/s relationships to burst out of the gate, but falter when life intervenes. I decided to write it anyway because my friend Elizabeth told me that much of the story is in the wanting itself, in the passion to pursue this scary, trembling feeling.

I am no easy conquest. I have my expectations born of Dominants who knew their stuff, I have my position in Rose & Thorn, and then there is my personality which ranges from Diva to Semi-Diva. It's more than most Dominants can handle, and who could blame them? My Dominant must be superior in his mind and heart; he must not be afraid of me even deep down where he thinks I cannot see.

For me to turn control over to him, I need to know he can say "no" to me. I need to believe it completely. Most Dominants cannot do this because my mind, my passion, and my drive are stronger than theirs. It's not because I have so much experience in BDSM, because in truth I don't, compared to many. I have had several long-term relationships with Dominants, but they were all of the "go out to dinner, come home and play, then go home" variety. While the passion was there, I knew whatever it was I was experiencing would be over in a few hours. Now, today, that is not enough.

There are Dominants whose experience is e-based: e-mail, chat rooms, phone calls. That is not enough for me. I need the presence of power over me; I need the comfort of his arms afterward when I cry. Other Dominants have played at a hundred play parties, flogging and paddling until the wee hours, but this is not sufficient either. I need privacy to let go, to allow my submission to soar light and free. Most of all, I need the connection, not just of someone able to tell me what to do and have me do it, but the relationship which makes those things meaningful.

I do not care if he owns a thousand dollars of floggers and whips and cuffs; rather he must have a mind who can see me, really see me. I care little about "play." I need connection. It is one thing to play with someone, but a whole other thing to truly turn it over.

As I wait and we negotiate, I flip from joy to fear. I do not go into this without trepidation. What will it be like to really belong to someone? Will I allow my fears to keep me from being genuinely present with him? Will I balk, struggle against his will? Or will I be able to finally rest, to settle into his hold with a gentle sigh?

If it is not him, it will be another. I have waited many months, even years, and I will wait longer if I have to. This time that dark magic will come by its own power, lifting me up and flying high over the trees of this mysterious and silent night.

A Week Later

I am a little over a week into negotiations with Tyler for a 24/7 relationship. Our discussions have stalled, leaving me with many questions, so many questions.

I have played in plenty of scenes, where a short negotiation to determine the general sway of things was sufficient. My Dominant would sit with me for a bit, ask about my boundaries, needs, fears, and the rest. What things have I not yet experienced but want to? What's on my NO list? What health issues do I have which might affect play? Where do I come into this emotionally? What do they want from me as a Submissive? I have been in a few longer-term relationships, where these same conversations stretched out for a few hours. These same questions loom even larger, and take even longer to process when it comes to the intense commitment of a 24/7 situation.

I'm pretty forthcoming about these things; I have no secrets. Usually the answers come easily, and we can always negotiate further as things come up. For every hour spent in play, there are two hours spent in life: cooking, cuddling, conversation. Plenty of time to process any new issues.

But with a 24/7 arrangement, things are so much grander. I must have sufficient trust and faith in this person to turn myself over to him completely–mind, body, heart. This intimacy is an entirely different beast than the here-or-there play. There is a greater emotional vulnerability, not just because of what I'm giving to him, but because I don't already know him well enough to know how he will handle the emotional part. And we all know the emotional part is the hard part.

I imagine a 24/7 negotiation will be a number of discussions over time, a flowering foundation which solidifies and deepens until we are ready to take the plunge. There are so many things to get out on the table before it all starts. After we are enmeshed, it will be harder to renegotiate. I don't want to be yanked in and out of subspace in order to figure out how the grocery bill will be handled or whether or not he can have another Submissive in the upstairs bedroom.

I have a few fears, but not many. I look at this as an opportunity to experience a transforming connection with myself, with him, and with my spirituality. My sex life is fairly negotiable, and in fact I have sampled many of the flavors of BDSM. But my economic life, my private life, my spiritual life are not negotiable. How will we work out a compromise in these areas which are so foundational to my life?

More importantly, will he know how to handle things when emotional issues come up, for they surely will. Is he grounded enough to manage not only his own feelings and needs, but mine, which will be so much more tender in this situation? With some of my autonomy given up, will I be able to distance myself emotionally if I need to? If I am confused and lost, will he be able to lead me out of the woods or will he opt out?

Tyler has his own fears; he is afraid I will fall in love with him. Is this born out of a fear that he cannot handle love? I have only fallen in love with one of my D/s partners in the eight years of being in the lifestyle, but even so I cannot give him any guarantee. Or can it be that Tyler is afraid of falling in love with me?

At this moment I am a wee bit infatuated with him, actually not him so much as with what he has to offer me. It's natural, I suppose, because this is the first time I've been so close to these fantasies coming true. But is that "love?" At 20, I might have confused infatuation with love, but not at 38. I wonder, if he is so afraid of love, does he have the emotional maturity to handle the Dominant responsibilities of a 24/7 relationship?"

I know there is a shadowy love-like realm when one is in a D/s relationship. The feeling of total trust and dependence which comes with deep submission can seem like love, I've felt it. But in the light of day I could always see it for what it was, a toss-up of lust, submission, and passion. If only there were a word for this transforming magic.

One of my Dominants, Ryan, understood this phenomenon. He understood the depth of Submissive vulnerability and dealt with the emotional pitfalls responsibly, as Submissives need from their Dominants. When he saw me teetering on the edge of falling for him, he'd sit me down, and have a gentle talk with me. Master Ryan knew himself, and in his knowing was unafraid of me or anything else.

Tyler is afraid that after the three-week 24/7 contract I will want more from him than he's prepared to give. But I wonder, isn't it natural to want an ongoing relationship with someone who has taken you to the deepest place? Would I want to go there with him even once, knowing that precisely at the three-week mark, everything may stop cold? Even if it was not love we had, but instead a caring commitment of another sort, wouldn't even that suppose some kind of ongoing conversation?

We started negotiations last week, but as of this writing there has been no meaningful communication for many days. Is he just plain thoughtless to leave me hanging? Is he paralyzed by the reality of negotiating? Has he gotten himself in too deep and now doesn't know how to proceed? I may never know. Regardless of the reason, do I want to risk myself for someone who cannot reach back to me when the going gets tough?

So, I'm guessing things will not go ahead. I'm guessing that while Tyler has two years of training as a Dominant, with paddling and bondage galore, in his heart he is not ready for something with such a strong emotional component as is central to a 24/7 engagement. I still don't know where this will end up, but I'm staying open to the possibilities. For now I will just be present to the limbo state of negotiation; after all... it has only been a week.

Postscript

I had hoped Tyler and I would be able to negotiate something workable, but soon I recognized our goals were not in alignment. Our beliefs about communication differ widely in that I believe communication is the foundation of any relationship, doubly so for the D/s persuasion. I can't say quite what Tyler's perspective is, but it is not the same as mine.

Nevertheless, our negotiation was successful in that we both discovered what we need to know about the other person. Although I didn't like Tyler's style of communication, I can't fault him for making different choices than I would. People often think a "negotiation" must lead to the desired goal to be a success, but in fact the negotiation is designed to provide sufficient information to make a decision. It's too bad I couldn't commit to any further play with him, but I do not regret having experienced this first negotiation, regardless of the outcome. And I will always appreciate the opportunity he gave me to get in touch with this deep desire.

Perhaps something else lies ahead for Tyler and me, but for the moment, this story is complete.

Just Call me a Bedroom Submissive

A Dominant once told me in a lofty tone of voice that I was "just a bedroom Submissive." At the time I was a bit offended, because I could tell he didn't have much respect for those "bedroom Submissives," whatever they were. In his world, I was not a true Submissive, and definitely not a true Slave. In his world, I wasn't much at all.

After getting over my pique at being called a name, I realized, well hell, he was right! My career, my writing, my financial life, my workouts, my relationships with my friends, even my relationship with God; all those things are mine and mine alone. What's left then? Yes the bedroom, that's what's left. My sexuality belongs to my Dominant, and that's what makes me a bedroom Submissive. That is no small thing however, and it is not the dregs of the rest of my life either. Rather, it is the cornerstone of my intimate identity, a huge gift for the right Dominant.

Why was it that Carson was looking down me for being a bedroom Submissive? Did he think that these things I wouldn't give up made me less committed somehow? Did he think I was not serious enough about BDSM? Or maybe, by doing it only in the figurative bedroom we were tip toeing a little too close to plain old vanilla sex. I love to quote my friend Gary Switch who said, "Yes, I admit it: we use BDSM as foreplay! You can kick us out of the lifestyle club, now. We'll go quietly." He's joking, and he's not. There is a hierarchy of "realness" in BDSM and silly as it may seem, there are people who would kick him out of the lifestyle club. He's in the dungeon of least respect there, along with the dabblers and weekend warriors.

Being a "Bedroom Submissive" isn't quite at the dank level that Gary resides in, but not far from it. On the other end of the spectrum are those who fancy themselves True Dominants and True Submissives, who live it 24/7 and dedicate their entire lives to BDSM. A little of this also has to do with a minority of BDSM purists who believe in keeping with puritanical and Christian beliefs, BDSM should be practiced without the sexual element. In contrast, I believe that sex magic is an undeniable and spiritual force on it's own, even more potent when in combination with scene play. What's important about that approach is not whether they are right or wrong, but in the limited way that they are approaching sexual energy.

What then is the truth of where I lay on the continuum? If you insist on labels, I draw myself somewhere in the middling ground. Because I am a writer and leader I get a certain level of validity that I might not have if I were simply practicing BDSM my own way in a less high profile way. I am far more than a weekend dabbler (although I respect them fully) but far less than Carson who has tens of thousands of dollars in BDSM equipment littering his home. It isn't just how much money and time he spends on this equipment, it's the fact that all his personal time is spent practicing BDSM technique and interacting with BDSM people. While this seems a bit over the top from my, eh hem, lofty

perspective, I nevertheless accord him the same respect as I give the weekend dabblers.
 This reflects the very real aspect of each of us measuring others using our own yardstick. To Carson, I am less of a Submissive because I wasn't submitting as much as he wanted me to, not unlike that saying that a slut is defined as someone who is getting more than you are. Carson was right about me being a bedroom Submissive, but not right that there's anything wrong with that. His need to put me down tells me more about his narrow frame of reference than it does about me. By my own Dominant's definition, I am a Submissive just fine. By my own definition, which is the most important one, I am exactly the right kind of Submissive. There is no "real" submission to measure up to. There is only who I am, which is just right for me.
 Name calling aside, what do I have to offer as a Submissive, as a real person? I have passion. I have a thoughtful and engaged mind. When I give it up I'm fully present. I know what I want and I'm willing and able to say so. I love sex, I love BDSM, and I am uninhibited. "Yes, I'll try that." Dominate me and you have Dominated something worthwhile.
 So where does that leave me? I will accept that title of being a bedroom Submissive, maybe even wave that flag outside my bedroom window. Or maybe I'll throw all those labels out the window and simply be myself. I'll do that because if I allowed Carson or anyone to tell me that my style of doing this lifestyle is less meaningful somehow, then I am allowing him to commit the worst of BDSM sins, and that is to disrespect our fellow travelers in their path. With the world being as it is, we need to support each other in every way we can, not tear each other down. So I say to Carson, and all the critics of the BDSM community: "Yes, I'm a bedroom Submissive; no, I'm not; and maybe I'm something else entirely."

Between Domspace and Subspace

One evening, a late and dark night in December, I was fucking the holy heck out of Moby when the strangest thing happened. Even as I took him like the piece of meat that he was, I felt my Domspace stealing over into Subspace. Even as I took him, there was a corner of my mind that was not taking, but being taken. It was a hazy moment born of my switchable nature. Fortunately, Moby didn't know this was happening to me, so I suppose what he didn't know didn't hurt him. But I wonder sometimes if this mental shift affected the dynamic of our relationship in ways that I might never know.

A similar thing happened with Griffin during our first scene together. Unlike Moby, Griffin is a Switch, and for this evening he was in Dominant mode. During the scene, he admitted that he had slipped into a Submissive headspace. This admission yanked me out of subspace, and worse, brought out my dominant side which probably didn't help things any. The experience wasn't any great shakes for Griffin either.

The next day when I talked to him about it, I explained the importance of deciding on a role and sticking with it, not to mention not telling your Submissive if you have a moment of that sort (or at least not admitting it during the scene). Because Griffin is also a novice, he is learning to control his focus in a scene, both by staying in a dominant frame of mind and also not getting distracted by the mechanics. Now that he's aware of this problem, I think he'll be able to manage it because he has experience in focusing his spiritual energy and because he is aware of several activities that put him in subspace by the simple act of doing them.

I haven't heard that many people talking about this particular issue; maybe because it might seem like the Dominant had failed somehow. But having observed this phenomenon both in myself as well as others, I think it's probably not all that uncommon. Other partners didn't always admit it as Griffin did, but I could see in their eyes the unmistakable expression of submission denied. I think it might have to do with switches who have a primary side to their switch personality. For example, I am 85% Submissive and 15% Dominant, which might explain my mind slipping into a Submissive headspace rather than the reverse. This is supported by the fact that the three Submissives I know who also experienced this were primarily submissive, dominating only as a sideline.

One of the things I've discovered is that some submissive men pretend to be dominant in order to attract a woman out of the relatively larger pool of submissive women. Sounds bizarre I know, but I think it's just a numbers thing, resulting in rather messy results as you can imagine. My way of dealing with this is to agree on a state of parity, where we take turns. With Griffin I could see that he would love to be submissive all of the time, but then so would I. With some partners it turned out that they really were unable to dominate on equal time, but I think that Griffin will be better able to access his Dominant side because of his experience with being a spiritual teacher, which has an undertone of dominance to it.

What is particularly attractive is Griffin's expertise as a spiritual guide, a shaman. I want this part of him very much, so I'm willing to help him to become a skilled Dominant in trade. Griffin has the potential to be a high caliber player because he has the spiritual thing already in place. He understands that there is a difference between just flogging someone as a physical exercise, and flogging as a way of transforming your energy to your Submissive. I have felt his energy through his hands, and I suspect that a flogger or whatever tool will be just another extension of his fingers.

It would be nice if our minds always did what we told them, which would help to prevent those mushy domspace/subspace things. Still, I think there may be some advantages to this flexibility of the mind. Switches obviously have twice the opportunities for partners, but there is also a natural balance to people with switch natures, which may give them a more grounded approach. Just as I am turned on by the androgynous in both men and women, I believe that the best players have experienced what it's like on both sides of the whip. For this broader field of experience and interest, I am willing to deal with the odd and sometimes unexpected oddities of the switch nature.

Vicarious Submission

    There are only a few men I've ever really loved, and Garrett was one of them. He had long silky hair, longer than mine, which cascaded over me when we made love. Being only 19, I sometimes got defensive about having to explain that long hair to my friends. Garrett said that he wasn't trying to make a statement, he just liked it that way. Of course back then hair was always a statement, but then there wasn't any rebellion in him so I believed it. The power of our connection branded that image into my consciousness, all the way through Moby, who would arrive in my life fifteen years later. Moby had that vulnerable something, a something which attracted both men and women and was perhaps inflamed by his long red hair which reflected sunlight as if he were an angel.

    I suppose that Moby's unique style got branded into me as well, because it was the red hair and gentle inclinations that drew me to Alice. The first thing I saw was morning sunshine shimmering off her wavy red locks. She too had that vulnerable something, the something that makes you want to cradle her in your arms, gently, carefully. Unlike me, Alice actually looks and acts like you might suppose a "real" Submissive to look like. She is shy and unlikely to take the stage as I do. Almost a little frightened really, like a butterfly touched down on your hand, but which is there for the grace of God, for a moment.

    My good friend Leela, an avowed lesbian, just couldn't figure it. Leela knows that I'm pretty much straight when it comes to affairs of the heart (or loins). I responded by quoting Woody Allen who said that bisexuality has the advantage because you get twice the chance of a date on Saturday night. No, I can't say I'd know exactly what to do with a girl, but I'm willing to find out. I have been with a few women bye the bye, but it never really clicked; maybe I'm just too phallo-centric. On the other hand, my relationships with women are far more peaceful and stable than most I've had with men. Maybe that phallo-centric thing translates into just plain too much trouble.

    In any case, I'm not one to cut someone out of the running just because they have the wrong equipment. I soon found myself fantasizing about Alice, not about holding her so gently actually, but about torturing her. Her body, curvy and delicate, is stretched tight with ropes. A blush rises from her belly to her neck, and her skin heats as the pain passes through my hands into her. Her eyes are dark and yearning, in that precarious place just between control and weeping. Another moment and her tears run down to the sheets as I hurt her, make her beg, make her cry.

    Or maybe we will be at a party. She will sit naked between my legs, my hands running along the undersides of her breasts, over her white skin. I spread her legs apart, hold them wide, so that others, strangers can put their fingers on her and in her. Sometimes I blindfold her so that she doesn't know whose fingers are sliding into her pussy or spreading apart her ass cheeks. Her trembling transfers to my body, but she doesn't fight it. She gives all of herself to me, open and helpless like a beautiful butterfly pinned to my mat.

    In a funny way, it's really me who wants to be pinned to that mat, helpless and fluttering. I who wish to have him open my legs and make me a toy. I want to do for her what I want done to me. And yet, while Submissives glom onto me left and right, Dominants are far harder to come by. What is it to explore submission vicariously, not through my own heightened senses but through those of another? Why has the universe brought such a strange thing into my life? Is it even fair to take her into those dark waters? Is this real, or will I resent her later after I have finally coaxed her into my sheets?

It's not just paranoid rambling on my part. When I finally convinced my friend Diego, a sometime Switch, to keep up the quid pro quo and dominate me, it turned out that he was more of a sometime Submissive than a sometime Switch. Even as he pulled and twisted my nipples sweetly, painfully; even as he talked to me in his low commanding voice; even with all this he yearned to be in my place. Oh yes, he wanted me to twist his nipples sweetly, painfully, talking in my own commanding tones. Diego could go through the motions all right, but his heart wasn't in it. It's the same when I'm dominant. I enjoy the accoutrements of the relationship: the trophy sub on my arm, charming conversation over a turkey dinner, the erotic massage afterward. But deep down, I want to be that Submissive, feeling just like Peter Pan when Tinkerbell holds his hand tightly and whispers "Fly, Fly!"

While I wait for my own Tinkerbell to take me on my next magical trip, will I spend my Friday evenings writing? Or will I be vicariously submissive, leaning down to nibble Alice's slender neck and then lower for a much deeper bite? Will it be enough to submit through her, even as she struggles against the ropes, against me, and then settles into my arms? Will it be enough even if my own heart isn't in it?

Part II - Unconventional Explorations

They say that we naturally assume that our upbringing was "normal," and I'd have to agree. It was only when I became an adult that I realized that my approach to life was quite unusual. My mother was a radical person, ahead of her time in many ways, but particularly in the sexual arena. Being a psychologist, she brought me up a la Rational Emotive Therapy, which she learned from the famed psychologist Dr. Albert Ellis (who I also revere). This section includes some writings that look at delicate and sometimes controversial topics.

Born a Hoochie Mama - and Where I Got Those Unconventional Ideas

One steamy summer night of my junior year in high school, I was hanging around one of those parties populated by the offbeat intellectuals of my high school set, the so-called "frisbee people." Ours was no friendly tossing-about-the-yard game however; rather a determined snap of a competition-sized Frisbee, whipped with all the energy of kids too smart for their own good. We weren't the only clique at this particular party and in the half darkness I observed a local jock. He was in a league foreign to my own, but still attractive for the cocky look in his eyes. I wanted to sleep with him and hesitated only a fraction of a second as I leaned close and whispered "I heard you're well-endowed." Of course he responded with "Would you like to find out?" And of course I did.

Even at sixteen I was aware of my own sexual precociousness. I "got" sex, and I knew that I got it. I understood how to flirt, how to seduce, how to make love. This came not from early sexual abuse as some might assume, but from a combination of my mother's razzy attitude and genetic poetry.

It may have been in the genes, but I didn't know it until maybe the realm of twelve years old when I had an unexpected urge to hump my bed headboard. The wooden curves bruised a bit, perhaps foretelling my future BDSM orientation. Fortunately it wasn't long after that I discovered my mother's electric vibrator, the glorious Prelude III. The sensations spoiled me sufficiently to disdain the hand job for life. Every afternoon I'd slip into her room to buzz out, and then spend the evening worrying she'd notice the vibrator was warm. Mom never did ask me about it though. I think she never noticed because despite not being shy about sexual matters, she sure wasn't any more observant than I am.

My mother was a radical and practical woman; a woman who not only believed sex is a joyous gift from God but who also left brochures on contraception in the bathroom. At fourteen I was as organized as I am now, and so visited Planned Parenthood a full year before I would ever have intercourse. I scribbled a shortlist of first-time candidates and decided on Daniel, a good friend although not technically a boyfriend. I chose him because his baseball-toned body glowed, setting off his sun-bleached hair. I wanted to always be able to say my first lover was a stud, and so I have. One afternoon I proposed that he be the recipient of my cherry, and he cheerfully accepted. He was probably thrilled at the direct approach. In order to score a blow job, Daniel insisted I go down on him because otherwise he'd suffer from blue balls, which was apparently medically threatening. Who would've thought I'd fall for that old line? In my defense it sounded daringly new the afternoon I lost my virginity. He never did go down on me though, and I didn't have the cojones, blue or otherwise, to call him on his hypocrisy. I would also discover a year later that he too had been a virgin, although admittedly I probably wouldn't have slept with him had I known.

Daniel and I did the hoochie every Wednesday at 3 PM for a year. Did I love him? No. Did I orgasm? No. Did I know that I was missing something? Yes. It wasn't love I missed, rather a

35

lover who could make me fly, one who'd make love to me at 2 AM on intermittent nights.

This lover came along in the form of Duncan, a chess-playing, frisbee-tossing geek, a geek with a strange charisma which kept me up nights obsessing over him, an obsession that would continue unabated through my college years. His hands were those of a magic man, electric with sensuality. Duncan worked part-time delivering for the local pharmacy, so I'd call for a box of cough drops every time I got itchy. Even years later, glimpsing a pale green van can induce me to arousal.

I've always approached relationships with this kind of ease, but the whole thing does seem more weighty for most young people, especially when they are taught that sex is a scary and secretive thing. One of the most damaging issues is the tendency to think of young women as sexual victims and of young men as sexual predators. In the article *The Sex Lives of Kid*s, Dennie Hughs writes, "we need to move away from the idea that girls who engage in oral sex but not intercourse are 'technical' virgins - that you're not having sex because no one's penetrating you. Let girls know that every time you do something like that, you compromise yourself and give up some of your power." It sounds like she's suggesting girls would give up less power if they just had the darn intercourse and stopped fooling around with labels. In fact she probably meant that whether it be oral sex or intercourse, women lose power when they have sex. She never mentions that boys might also lose power by sleeping with someone, or that both girls or boys might suffer emotionally when they have sex for the wrong reasons.

Is it not possible that girls could be "gaining" power by having sex? Even possible that sex not be about power at all? If a girl is a victim to start with, she may be well be victimized by someone's sexual agenda. Victimization is about low self esteem, not about sex. She can equally be

36

emotionally or physically victimized by an abusive partner. And yet it would be foolish to tell young people to abstain from relationships, because it is the relationship dynamic which creates the atmosphere where we can develop interaction skills.

In contrast, a budding bawdy girl like myself may be empowered by the sexual experience. Even as a Submissive in a BDSM relationship, I am "exchanging" power with my Dominant, not "giving up" anything. I am still a whole person, with or without a Dominant.

In this same article, co-author Dr. Drew Pinsky states, "deep feelings of intimacy are overwhelming and confusing and can easily be exploited and most experts believe that kids under 16 do not have the psychological or neurological development necessary to satisfactorily manage these feelings." Although Dr. Drew may not have been correct about me personally, many young people are clearly not ready to handle the complexities of sexual relations. This being the case, why not provide young people with both emotional and sexual skills to navigate relationships?

My mother provided me with navigation, although unconventional to be sure. She never told me to keep my knees together or not to sleep around. She never told me that monogamy is the only option, or to wait until marriage to make love. Good thing, because I never did marry and if I'd waited I'd still be a virgin at nearly 40.

Instead, she told me the story about how she made love the first time with her uncle, a consensual and loving experience. She explained that most people have a series of love relationships in their lives, and that it's okay to accept this as a natural circumstance. She said sometimes the best lovers were not the best looking ones, and that just because you loved someone, they might not be a good partner for you. Somewhere in my college years, she told me about the open relationship she and my father had and how they worked out the rules. And then there were those brochures in the bathroom.

    My mother may not have given me much in the way of traditional relationship advice, but she did teach me to make my own decisions. Her advice made losing my virginity at fifteen an exciting and decisive experience. I have enjoyed a number of open relationships without the destruction jealousy brings. I never felt pressured to have children, and so have been free to explore my creative energy without encumbrances.

    When I reach sixty I will become the eccentric aunt archetype: artsy and a bit eccentric. I will wear short skirts with hot pink aerobic shoes, and speak my mind when I've a mind to. I will have a lover or two, and flirt with sexy Italian men serving me New York Style pizza. I will have been a bawdy girl and a hoochie mama and regretted nothing. I may not have the things every little girl was brought up to think she should have, but I will have had a life defined by my own vision.

Fat Women, Body Image, And Sexual Politics In The BDSM Scene

My name is Sadie and I'm fat. That is, fat and beautiful. Zaftig. Rubenesque. Soft and cuddly, and really fun to hug. I am a size 24, and in general, if you don't like it, you can lump it. It helps that I am also in fabulous shape with calves of steel and six pack abs (which can't be seen under my tummy, but I know they're there)

This is a little bit about me and a lot about everyone who has body image issues. It's a lot about women, and a little about men. It's about how I came to love my body, and also how body image and self-esteem function in the D/s context. When I started thinking about writing this piece, I wasn't sure if I had anything useful to say. After all, as my friend Elizabeth told me "you have the best body image of anyone I know, thin or fat."

The story of how I got here doesn't have a lot to do with BDSM, so I won't go into excess detail. Suffice it to say that once upon a time I was addicted to food and hated my body. In my mid 20's I went to Overeaters Anonymous and made friends with Nicole, another addict who happened to be a size five, but who also ate her chicken pot pies half frozen because she couldn't wait for them to bake fully. She was also one hell of a snappy dresser. Nicole taught me that self-hatred is an equal opportunity force of destruction for both fat and thin women, not to mention how to be one hell of a snappy dresser.

Is The BDSM Scene Any Different Than Vanilla Life?

Some years later I entered the BDSM lifestyle pretty much at peace with those issues. I don't have any research basis for this, but there does seem to be more plus-sized women in the scene. Perhaps they are attracted in greater numbers because their size is less of an issue than what they have to offer through their submission or their domination.

The scene offers some wonderful things that the vanilla world does not. The biggest one is that due to numbers alone, way more men than women, I could have been a complete ass, a total bitch, or a whining doormat and I still would have had no shortage of Dominants a'knocking at my door. While I have never found it particularly difficult to find lovers in the vanilla world, in the BDSM world they're lined up on the doorstep. Before Vermont even had a D/s community, I posted a personals ad in alt.personals.bondage and over a few years met and went out with no less than 40 Dominants. Is this because I'm God's gift to men? As much as I'd like to think so, it's unlikely. There some are very real differences which account for this phenomenon.

While we come from all walks of life, BDSMers all have a love for the alternative. We are not people who spend every Wednesday night engaged in military-style intercourse. We love passion, the power exchange, and the magic of sexual self-expression. This attitude translates, generally speaking, into a more open-minded attitude toward size, not to mention age, gender, race, and orientation. When I look for a Dominant, I'm looking less at his career path, and more for his ability to know himself and control me. When I look for a Submissive, I'm looking less for his economic viability, and more for his capacity to be vulnerable, for his emotional stability. Looks are nice, and heaven knows I like to have a hot trophy Submissive hanging on my leash, but the bottom line is that after a scene, I want to be able to connect with this person on a deeper level. After the party, I want to be able to cuddle up with them over a bowl of popcorn and watch Arsenic and Old Lace.

Unlike our vanilla friends who rarely see large naked bodies, we have many opportunities through play parties and demos to look at, get used to, and eventually admire the soft curves of fat people. It is at first astounding, and then liberating to see a large man or woman walk around a play party stark naked, proud of their body, fully loved. It's hard not to like someone who likes herself so much.

How To Get Over It

The thing about body issues is that everyone has them, women and men, thin and fat, you and me. After all, if I never had any body issues, the world would not need me to be an activist for size acceptance. If you want to get over self-criticism, here are some things you can try. Start by communicating with your body, using affirmations to find the beautiful parts about yourself, not just physically, but emotionally and spiritually. Listen to what your body has to say, and respect your own path. This is the foundation of self-love. If you love yourself, loving your body will follow.

On the practical side, go to some play parties or other public situations where you will be able to observe people of all sizes and shapes enjoying themselves. Replace any critical thoughts in your head with positive ones about the beauty of their bodies, whether it be good skin, soft curves, great butt to spank, strong muscles, or wonderful handfuls of breasts. Talk to your friends about what beautiful thing you saw in this larger person. If it's not a physical attribute, notice their courage for playing in public, their love of their own body, or their unself-consciousness. For the female Dominant, size can be an advantage, projecting a powerful physical presence which attracts Submissives. If you have this advantage, use it.

Invite some friends over and do a little play under more controlled conditions. You'll be able to see how it feels to share your fears with people you trust. Here again, you don't need to bare it all. Think about the parts of your body you like best and start with those. For example, I feel most confident about my breasts, waist and legs. So when I first played in public I wore a short skirt, but bared the rest of me. When I played with one Submissive who was shy about his tummy (he wasn't fat, but he didn't work out and was a bit soft there), I had him bare his ass and penis, both very fine, but allowed him to wear a tank top. Showing this kind of love and care for his feelings also helped him to come to terms with his body.

I found I felt more confident when my friends and/or play partners were also plus-sized. Over time I discovered play partners who weren't fat themselves, but who appreciated my body nevertheless for its strength, flexibility, health, and energy.

When you are ready, consider doing some public play at a party. You do not have to go whole hog and strut around nekkid. Take some trusted friends along and give it a try.

Work out! There is nothing like the confidence and strength that comes from being in good shape. While we should all be respected regardless of our size, it's much harder for people to criticize me knowing that 1. I'm in better shape than they are, and that 2. I can kick their butt.

Wear sexy clothes. The best part about Scene parties is the opportunity to dress like a slut. Scene events are one of the few places where you can wear revealing, sexy, exotic clothing, and have it be appreciated. Show off your best attribute. Have you ever seen me in a high necked shirt or a long skirt? Looking good translates to feeling good. Dress not because you feel you should, but because showing off your body will increase your confidence. Also known as fake it till you make it. Lastly – if you like yourself and your body – act like it. Talk about body image to your friends. Dress well. Take care of your body. Be a role model.

The Big Picture
This is my theory about men and body size:

25% Love Plus Sized Women Like Me! One vanilla, but aggressive lover in the midst of fucking my brains out, whispered "those guys who like skinny women don't know what they're missing!" A New Hampshire Dominant says, "I prefer larger Submissives. There's more flesh to play with and I don't have to worry so much about hitting bones." Another scene player says "Personally, I find the sight of a voluptuous woman bound tightly much more stirring than a slim woman. It is much more gratifying to spank a well-rounded bottom than a skinny one."
25% Do Not Notice Body Size At All. One Dominant said to me, "I get so irritated with these Submissives who talk about and criticize their bodies all the time. It makes me focus on the negative things about them, and to be honest, I really just do not care about whether or not they have a tummy or not, or have big thighs or not, or whatever. I just don't look at people that way."
25% Prefer Slimmer Woman, But Are Open To Loving People For Who They Are, Not What They Look Like. Another Dominant said to me "I've been with big women and small women and it doesn't matter what size they are, so much as their personality and whether or not they're fun to be with in and out of bed."

25% Only Date Thin Women. One Submissive said about her partner "Recently as we were walking with our arms about each other, he commented 'the world is backwards.' He does not like the fact that I am not small enough to throw around the bed the way he would like."

100% of them are irritated by women who harp on their bodies and constantly put themselves down.

I know three Dominants who only get involved with thin women. Does it irk me? You bet it does, and at some level it limits our friendship. I need to know that my friends celebrate me in the same way I celebrate myself. I'm not saying each of us shouldn't be allowed to have our preferences, but to insist on one particular body type seems childish and closed-minded to me. I also don't go out with men who only date plus-sized women. That's just as ridiculous. I choose my men for their ability to be emotionally grounded, spiritually present, and engaged with life.

In any case, I'm still left with 75% of the men, so I say to hell with the ones who are stuck on size. In addition to my fat self, my zaftig self, my Rubenesque self, I am so much more. I am passion, joy, and spirituality. I am strength and weakness, Dominance and submission, taking and yielding. I am a whole person first, a fat woman second, and, I am really fun to hug.

The Nature of Sadism and the Sadism of My Nature

One night my Submissive, Moby, knelt before me in that position some call the slave position: knees spread wide, pelvis thrust forward, hands on his thighs, palms up. I loved seeing him this way, open to me, vulnerable to me. I ran my red crop up his legs, watched him tremble. I laid into him, into his ass, his balls, his most sensitive thighs until he couldn't take another blow, not one. Then I gave him what I call the "false choice" after which I switched to another pain, not the pounding sting of a crop, but the sweet torture, the deep torture of nipple clamps. Slow pain, twisted and burning, the kind which didn't even have a moment, the rush of cool air between each slice of the crop. When he couldn't take the nipple torture any more, he'd say so, and I'd switch back to the terrible crop. His need to suffer for me, his joy in turning over every bit of his body to me, his passion and pain and presence were all there in his eyes, dark and shining.

His "false choice" was that he chose to end one pain, but there was the other waiting there in the shadows. Which was worse? Which was better? The sudden sharp twang or the slow burn? How much longer could he take it, knowing no real relief was coming, even though he had the choice of when to stop. I was merciless, and another pain would be patiently waiting for him. I laid my head on the pillow and gazed up at his face, fixed upon mine. He was doing this for me, and he knew it. I knew it. And I loved torturing him. I like to make boys cry. I know it's hard for them. I felt powerful, indulgent, controlling, gleeful.

Later on when he rested in my arms, lost in the safety of my hold, I considered my sadistic nature. How could I be this way? Was this really me? I don't kill spiders, would never hit a child, would never hurt even Moby in any real, soulful way. But it is true, I am undeniably a sadist.

So many people in the D/s scene say I like this play or that, but "no pain." They want to stick with BDSM Lite: silk scarves tied to the bed, a little feather tease, maybe a little over-the-knee spanking. But no, no serious pain. Never struggling, suffering, weeping until all other things are forgotten.

I think I might have been that way too, long ago. That light version of things was like a light, fruity wine, sipped after a tinkle of glasses meeting in a toast after the play was over. Now I've had my taste of blood, and can only drink the dark, strong cordials of a darker, stronger experience. I want to give it, and I want to receive it, because I am a pain slut myself, wanting him to push me more and more and more until I am pushed right over, soaring into the chasm.

Some people think pain is when you twist an ankle, or burn a finger, but pain in the D/s context is hardly pain at all. I know this when I give, and when I receive. When I submit, pain transforms to a river of sensation, powerful as it swirls around my ankles, rising slowly, slowly until it engulfs my body. I love to suffer for him because I know in this one place, in this one act where I have given fully, my Dominant receives fully. I serve him by accepting, and myself by allowing myself to go as far as he will take me. I am tethered by his hand,

stayed in this place and distance from the outside world, until he returns me.
   Does the fact that I have this nature "mean" anything about who I am? Does it take away from my humanity... or possibly add to it? Can there be respect for something which seems on the surface to have no reason, no rationale, only pathological weirdness? Can I be a spiritual person as I am, committed to my spiritual path and still make sense of my enjoyment of Moby's pain, or even my own pain? How can this be reconciled with the other parts of me, the parts where I cuddle my cat, take food to the food bank, and call my sister every week?
   What if we were to bring sadism out in the open, to be discussed as easily as who won last night's hockey game? Would people only be able to liken me to a child abuser or someone who abuses her spouse? Probably so, but oh how wrong they'd be. Why aren't we allowed to talk about sadism? Why does it always go hand in hand with non-consensual acts? Is sadism by its very nature non-consensual? Or maybe this is just semantics, and at the crux of things lies some mysterious something. Something I feel while hurting, while being hurt; something that just needs another name?
   In our culture there is no regular Jane: the happy healthy sadist. Some think it's pathological to want to hurt someone, yet we all do it when we are grievously hurt or betrayed, rushing to hurt back, usually in the emotional realm. How easy it is to push the buttons of the people you love. How many times has a friend given me the silent treatment or said something cutting to hurt me. It may not be a whip, but that, too, is sadism.
   Perhaps humiliation is the mental side of sadism. I have not yet been humiliated by any Dominant, but maybe it's because none of my Dominants had that particular bent. Maybe it's that I just have an irrepressible sense of humor, or that some kind of religion or familial guilt is

necessary to induce true shame. Even when one Dominant urinated on me, all I felt was damp and sticky. My thoughts ran more toward taking a shower, not glorying in any humiliation. My rational mind knew urine is pure, pure enough to drink, not to mention useful to people dying on the desert sands. Too practical I know, and I digress.

Maybe I need something stronger than a little piss. My friend Brandon wrote something in his personals ad which made me think if anyone could, he could humiliate me. He wrote about making his Submissives rub their cunts on his leg, hump his leg, and beg to be allowed to come. I could see myself, desperate after weeks of being denied sexual release, awkwardly trying to rub myself enough to get off. I would be so needy to be touched, to be allowed a tiny bit of pleasure, that I would beg him. Yes, begging would be humiliating. I knew he would like seeing me reduced by his ownership of my sexuality. This is something I've always wanted, not the begging for the orgasm, but the fact of no longer being in control of my own sexuality. Surrender doesn't get any deeper.

Is this sadism of the mental kind? Maybe. Would it be consensual on both our parts? Of course. If sadism is consensual, is it still sadism? Or does the willingness, even eagerness of the participants somehow morph it into something else, a horse of a different color? What is that color? Is it as false a choice as I gave Moby, or something as deep and dark and sweet as the cordial I can still taste on my lips?

Meeting the Devil at the Crossroads of Spirituality, Sexuality, Love, and BDSM

When you sleep with someone, your body makes a promise whether you do or not.
~ Julie (Cameron Diaz) in the movie *Vanilla Sky*

    Back in high school there was a clear delineation between what was Sex and what was Not. We knew this because we all listened to Meatloaf's eight minute make-out song "Paradise by the Dashboard Light." Under the music and under our moans, the baseball commentator made it perfectly clear that he may have gotten in a few gropes, but that the home run Just Wasn't Gonna Happen.
    We all knew, in some cultural/genetic way, that kissing was first base; above the belt was second, and below, third. Intercourse, of course, was the home run. My friends didn't ask me whether my experience was fulfilling emotionally, they asked me if I made a home run. They wanted to know if I had Had Sex (intercourse) or Didn't (anything else). And they weren't asking about anal sex, oral sex, or God knows what other orifice sex. They were talking about good old missionary vaginal sex.

Of course, even sexually unsophisticated adults know there's a whole world between licking your lips for the first kiss and taking a drag from the post-coital cigarette. Even as a foolish teenager, we gals should have been asking not whether you fucked (which was nice) but whether you came (which was real nice). Much easier for guys, since they get one with the other for the most part by definition.

Now that I'm scuba diving in the waters of D/s, things have gotten a bit more complex. In the beginning, I had some confusing moments describing my relationships to my friends. I didn't actually have intercourse with some of my partners, so did they count as lovers? By Meatloaf's assessment, I guess they didn't, but then my partner Bailey offered another option. He suggested I reframe how I defined sex, making love, and BDSM play. I ended up with a bunch of lists which kind of suggests I had gobs of lovers. Compared to some, I suppose I have. But from my perspective, I've never really had as much sex as I wanted, no matter how you define it.

On the love side, there's the list of men I loved who didn't love me (unrequited love). There's the men I didn't love, who loved me (a totally different list, unfortunately). There's the list of Real Lovers, guys I loved, who loved me back (a much shorter list).

On the sex side, there are the lovers, most of whom I didn't love, a few of whom I did, and some one-night-stands for color. There are one or two threesomes and a couple with women. There's the BDSM play with sex, and the BDSM play without sex, not to mention the BDSM play with love, and without.

Then there was the moment when Miguel kissed me after the fair, with lips tasting of maple cotton candy, and made me want to get on my knees, right there in the parking lot. But the kiss was all I got; I never saw the guy again. Does it have to be an overt dominant act to count? Or is it

50

enough that he took me there, even in a moment which melted as fast as cotton candy on my tongue?

My mother taught me that my body is a temple. She was talking in terms of eating a lot of whole wheat bread, I'm guessing, but I think she also believed that when you made love, there was a holy blending of the body and spirit. Being of the eastern way of spirituality, I believe the mind, body and soul are one. My friend Elizabeth says the same thing, that when you have sex, there's an elemental and entwining exchange of energy at the spiritual level which remains long after the physical act is finished.

I figure she's right, as long as it's "making love" we're talking about here. I've had mind-bogglingly good sex with guys I knew, and with some I barely knew. I've had lovers for years I never loved, but who I had a darn fine time with. I've made love with a few who loved me back, and who may not have been the fuck of all time, but who had something magic.

Then there's all those same permutations for my D/s partners. Only with Moby did our souls meet on the love, sex, and D/s levels. It was more than just an exchange of magic; it was the most astounding experience of my life. The rough thing about having had a soulmate like him is that it's a hard act to follow. I've been to the gourmet eight-course meal, with a different wine for each course. I've had the dessert afterward, a dark chocolate cake melting on my fork and in my mouth. How will I go back to fast food?

It's for those reasons I'm generally celibate these days. I haven't been able to reconcile fuck-buddies with the gourmet meal. Maybe I've been spoiled forever. This watershed changed my mind about sex and love, and I can only hope I'll find it like that again. I might not, but I hope I never regret it.

I also realized that it's not about which list you put your relationship on. I know a lot of scene people who only do sexually oriented play, others who only don't. A lot of them seem to think the label is important in itself; as if being a purist was a point of pride. I read about how in Mexico there is still a strong cultural value on virginity in young girls (why not young boys?). So the girls have oral sex, anal sex, God knows what other kind of sex. Somehow, because they don't have vaginal sex, they're still virgins. It's the Bill Clinton definition of sex, the one that everyone except Bill knew was bullshit.

It's not about which orifice you use so you can pretend you aren't having sex. It's not even about whether you actually have intercourse involving a penis and vagina, or whether you use your tongue and their ass. It's not whether you actually tied someone to the bed and flogged them, or if you just whispered it in their ear.

It's all intimacy.

Define it how you want, but the erotic tension is in there somewhere, a strand as delicate as a filament or as powerful as a cable. Even so, it's only partly about the sex. What it's really about is intimacy, which covers all those lists and whatever new ones I come up with.

So when I tell you I don't do casual play, it's not just about whether I want to go to first base, second base, or whatever. It's really about the next time I go play baseball of any kind, it'll be the kind where I can feel his presence even before he touches me. The kind where my heart rests softly in his arms. Where I can give up my power for a little while or longer, even if it's only as long as an eight minute make-out song.

Adultery, Betrayal, and How I Rationalized My Way Out of Things

Back in my vanilla days, I got hit on now and then by married men. No one actually said "my wife doesn't understand me," but the sentiment was there. I ran into Mark my first summer in Vermont while getting my motorcycle tuned up after a long winter's rest. Mark was big and muscled with grease under his fingernails, one of those rough and tough guys. He made a special visit out to my place to bring me a motorcycle part, and we ended up smooching in the grass, still damp from an afternoon rain. His roughened fingers raked my back, making me squeal even as he pulled up my bra and cradled my breasts. Did I know he was married? Yes I did. Did I have an excuse? No I did not. I was hot and he was hot and that was all we needed. He never called me again, which was a good thing. I was pretty darn close to sleeping with a married man, maybe the closest I've ever been.

My next brush with adultery happened when my friend Morelli fell in love with me. Of course, he was married to a shrew; no man trying to seduce you is ever married to an angel. We met in the downtown Burlington cemetery to consider our options. I liked him plenty, oh yes, because of his powerful body and his tender mind. There is a special attraction to someone being in love with you, no risk, no worries about rejection. But this time the specter of his wife was clearly in my line of sight. It was a close call, but I managed to leave, having given up just a few soulful kisses. I never heard from Morelli again, even after their divorce. His passion must have been more about escapism than it was about me.

A few years later my buddy Shawn, a Submissive with a taste for exhibitionism, asked me to watch him masturbate. Hmm, I thought, as long as I don't touch him, then he's not cheating on his wife and so neither am I. Shawn had a toned body, lithe and tanned, one which slipped into quite a few of my nighttime fantasies. So I watched as he stood on the back porch in the June sunshine where he might just be seen. No... I didn't touch him. I didn't feel so bad about this one, but then I didn't feel really good either. I couldn't help but wonder where that line was, and if I had crossed it.

It wasn't long after when I met friend Ken, a cross-dressing Submissive. He convinced me with soft and pleading words that I was the only person who he felt safe enough to come out to. He convinced me that this wasn't cheating because his wife didn't "do" BDSM and so therefore he had no choice but to get it elsewhere. I hadn't had a Submissive all to myself before, and I admit it stroked my ego to have someone choose me as his first. I gave in, engaging in one dinner with a flirtation chaser, one introductory scene with minimal skin contact, and one real scene where he freaked out and left five minutes after I told him to strip. No apology no explanation, so I thought I'd done some terrible thing. In any case, I rationalized that since we had barely touched, this really wasn't cheating. I wasn't actually party to adultery. I wasn't guilty of hurting some woman out there whom I never met. I wasn't responsible. Now I know it wasn't that I committed some horrific Dominant faux pas, but rather that the universe didn't want me messing with a married man.

This was the last time I ever considered a relationship with someone who was cheating on his partner (as opposed to a consensual open relationship). It's harder in the BDSM community to hold this line because so many married people need to express their orientation, but will not or cannot tell their partners. I don't have any answers for them, only my own choices to do or not to do. Being "party" to adultery is the same as adultery. You don't get dispensation from being one degree away.

I formally apologize to the four women I have disrespected through my selfish acts. I don't know your names, but I hope you will accept my apology, anyway.

The reality is that adultery is the same whether it is vanilla or D/s. The crux of the thing is not whether or not specific acts came into play, but the fact of our intimacy and the betrayal it caused. That's the sin. Those men betrayed the affection and trust of their wives, and I helped. For what it's worth, I won't do it again. The most important thing I own is my integrity, and that, at least, is intact from here on in.

Strong Female Submissives

If I had a nickel for every Submissive who hit on me, I could open my own dungeon. The real bummer about the whole thing is that I'm submissive myself. Oh sure, I top now and then, but when it comes down to it, my D/s orientation is submissive. So, you ask, why are Submissives glomming onto me like those alien pancakes glommed onto the officers of the Star Trek Enterprise? The answer is easy: it's my dominant personae. It starts with being a plus-sized woman, one who wears sexy and dramatic clothing. It continues with my articulate mind, my direct way of speaking, and my forwardness in asking for what I want.

Yet that person, the public person, is not my sexual orientation. I say orientation in the sense that I've committed myself to the lifestyle and no longer date 'nilla guys. When it comes to the bedroom, I love to serve. I love to be taken. I love to suffer. I love it all.

So why's it so hard to believe?

We've all seen media images of the powerful male executive who sees a mistress on the side. We understand that men like this need some time to let go, to not be in charge. Yet we never see media images of the powerful female executive slipping out for a quick bondage session, although the housewife donning a black latex catsuit to whip up a few afternoon callers is common enough. These are roles with which we're all familiar, the successful male executive and the housewife. These are roles which don't make any waves in our patriarchal culture, at least in public where it counts. You'd think in a culture which teaches women to give up their own needs for others, the obvious rebellion would be to go Dominant, but the obvious is not always the reality.

The dynamics of who we are in the bedroom, broadly speaking, versus who we are as people are circuitous. Just as the mind, soul, and body are all intertwined, so is our sexual orientation intertwined with who we are as a whole person. Yet it does not automatically follow they should present the same. If that were so, then we would all be exactly as we appear. We would no longer have our humanity of equal parts art and soul. Why should a person submissive in the bedroom be assumed to also submit in life? There's no obvious rationale to this statement, yet it's so commonly asked of me I have to believe that people cannot understand the difference between sexual orientation and personhood. The corollary is that Dominants, usually men, often assume I will submit to them simply because they are a Master, even though they are not my Master. Is this arrogance or just inexperience? Is it simpleminded and simpleheaded, or simply ignorant?

On the broader level for both men and women, there is often a confusion between submission and passivity. Being submissive doesn't mean you let people take advantage of you. In fact, having a strong self means you have more to give a Dominant. If you are nothing, if you are a doormat, there's no challenge or excitement in dominating you. Being a doormat is not an act of submission, but rather a state of helplessness which invites abuse.

I am a Submissive, which is a proactive choice of seeking to please my partner. He, in an equally proactive way, gives me the control and care I need. It's an equal exchange, so unlike the vanilla world where women are often taken for granted.

One of the wonderful differences in the D/s community is that the Submissive, female or male, may well bring home the bacon as well as fry it up in a pan, but because the exchange is a negotiated agreement, her contributions are fully appreciated and taken into consideration. This is not the assumption of the traditional family dynamic where women are often working full-time and have to come home to care for the home and children, with little help from their partners.

Generally speaking, both female and male Dominants carry the trait of dominance in their sexual orientation as well as in their lives. While the image of the successful male executive who is submissive may be a popular stereotype, I don't actually know any men like this. In fact, my experience with these men is that they tend to also be submissive in a broader sense. However I've been told quite a few times that my experience in this is not typical.

The interesting dynamic arises with submissive women. About half of us are like me, powerful energetic women who love to submit. The other half, or so, are submissive in all areas of their lives, quite often even passive.

What does this gender difference mean? I'm guessing the traditions of women's roles in our culture particularly affect those of us who are submissive sexually. Many of us struggle with wanting to express this side of ourselves without losing the independence for which our foremothers fought. We recognize that feminism is threatened by women who claim their sexual nature. Of course we don't want to lose what history has given us: freedom to vote, to work, and to make our own choices. Real feminism is about freedom to choose, which includes choosing our orientation.

We must educate both our sisters and our vanilla brethren that being submissive does not necessarily diminish our strength as women, individually or collectively. It is only when we become passive that we are truly diminished.
    On the most superficial level I, too, am that executive woman. I make decisions all day; I don't want to make them in the bedroom. One of the downsides of being a strong woman is that people figure you don't need attention or nurturing, but they could not be more wrong. In fact, because we receive less, we actually need it more than most. Being submissive allows me to accept the nurturing I need, that everyone needs.
    Part of this nurturing is being the center of attention. This person, this Dominant has spent time, money, and energy planning a scene designed just for me. It is so focused on me that he may not even orgasm, and is entirely understanding when I do the classic obnoxious lover's move of rolling over and falling asleep after the scene. On the surface, the classic scene is enacted by the Dominant, but at the foundation it's about taking the Submissive into a different headspace. Hackneyed as the phrase has become, it also comes down to the Submissive being ultimately in control. I give up my power within a certain sphere of influence, but even then, even at the very last minute I can make it all stop anytime by simply speaking my safeword.
    On a deeper level, serving is a spiritual act. Although I'm not a Christian, I like the story about how Jesus washed his follower's feet. In serving another, I put my self aside. My demanding, selfish, childish self. The self who wants what I want when I want it. For those few minutes of serving, I am lifted above my mundane wants. When I am free to fully express this side of myself, my submissive side, then I become even more of the strong woman I am outside the bedroom, the strong woman who revels both in her strength and in her submission.

The Submissive in Charge

Who's ultimately in control? The Submissive is, of course!

We've all heard this line bandied about, but does it make sense? Anyone can see that during a scene, the Dominant is clearly the one in charge, so it can't be about that. Submitting is predicated on giving up that control. If the Submissive were actually controlling the scene, they wouldn't by definition be submitting. So what's this catchphrase really mean?

There are two different kinds of control, control over the bottom line (the ultimate), and control over a particular sphere of influence. Being ultimately in control means that the Submissive can always use his safeword and stop the action; they have veto power. Veto power is an "if all else fails" measure, and not the same thing as being in control, however. Not the same thing at all.

The sphere of influence control refers to the areas that the two people have negotiated between them as the areas where the Dominant has freedom to act. Within this area he or she has a great deal of freedom, while respecting agreed-upon boundaries. This sphere covers quite a lot of area, and can be narrow as in a short scene in public or comprehensive as in the case of a Master/slave relationship, where all the slave's activities are under the Master's dominion. Of course the Submissive can always walk out that door, but barring that extremity, the Master makes the decisions.

Because of the broadness of the BDSM experience, I do not recommend the use of one safeword but rather the Green-Yellow-Red* system of communicating. This system allows for ongoing and easy-to-remember communication, which in most cases is preferable. This system is better because pushing someone all the way to a single safeword can be hurtful both physically and psychologically, particularly with a novice Submissive who may not know where their safeword lies. They may suffer a great deal in the period just before and after they safeword, pain which is unnecessary and can be easily prevented.

The other challenge with one safeword is that some Submissives have a hard time using their safeword at all. They might be worried that they will disappoint their Dominant, or they might have a personal goal to take as much as they can, even if it's not healthy for them. They may well not have a good idea where their endpoint is, or they may not be able to effectively judge because of the endorphins bopping around in their system.

I experienced this kind of repressed safewording with my Submissive Moby. A sister Dominant and I had organized a birthday scene for him, tying him up and torturing him deliciously. At one point she decided to put clothespins on his penis. I had put clothespins on his balls (on the skin) before, but not on his penis. Still, I figured he'd let us know if there was a problem. It wasn't until later that evening that I discovered that this act was well past his boundaries, and in fact had pretty much freaked him out. I was frustrated because he hadn't communicated this to me during the scene. This is a classic situation where Moby had the responsibility to express his feelings to me, and didn't. It turned out that he thought I'd be pleased with his ability to take the pain, and it didn't occur to him that I'd be upset about him not being true to his own needs, not to mention not communicating with me.

One Submissive I know told me, "I take the personal responsibility theory myself. I am in control of and responsible for myself, my physical and emotional well being. If I choose to allow another person to take over control of something in my life, then the outcome is still my responsibility. If it works out badly, then it's my fault for choosing the wrong person to assume control over those things which I have given up control over." This is an interesting approach, and definitely is something only for Submissives who are very self aware and competent.

There is also a question about whether a person in subspace has enough mental awareness and self control to safeword if they need to. I have found that for myself, no matter how deep into subspace I am, I am always fully able to safeword if needed. For many Submissives however, the mind-altering drug of subspace is so intense as to make rational thought impossible. Some might even argue that some experiences of subspace preclude rational thought by definition. For this reason, Dominants must be doubly careful. Fortunately for many, hard limits are instinctive and present themselves even under duress.

In the reverse situation, one of my Dominants once told me that he was going to push me all the way to safeword. He wanted to know exactly where that place was, and he also wanted me to learn how to say it, that it was okay to safeword. He knew that once I'd said the word the first time, it would be easier to say it in the future. He also recognized that this process made me conscious of actually going to safeword, and gave me a "muscle memory" of the experience of doing so. In another scene at another time, I might have been hard pressed to safeword perhaps because of physical or emotional stresses. Having done it the one time was educational and healthy for both of us.

Let me also add that I have never used my safeword with the majority of Dominants whom I have played with. Most of them are able to judge my state, and in fact can hear it in the change of tone in my voice in the way I say "ow!" Using the Green - Yellow - Red system has always provided sufficient information to prevent our ever getting to Red unintentionally. But not all Dominants are this observant, and especially if they are novices themselves they may be caught up with flogging technique or whatever.

One Dominant told me that he'd play with me until I safeworded (if I did) but if that occurred, play would cease immediately for the evening and he'd leave. I immediately recognized this approach for the dirty manipulation that it was, and I refused to get involved with him. What he didn't understand was when a person is pushed to the point of safewording, they may well need emotional love and care afterward. To push someone to their most extreme space and then to withdraw is the ultimate in irresponsible Domly behavior. It was almost a threat in that if I were to safeword, or in other words say "No" to him, then he would refuse to continue. What this says to me is that he wanted total submission without limits. That may be something you would negotiate with a long-time committed partner, but absolutely not with a new Submissive.

In contrast, you will also see some Submissives who think of their safeword as a technique to stop things they don't like, as opposed to using it strictly as an expression of having gone too far. In this scenario, the Submissive is indeed topping from the bottom, using the safeword to get their way. When you describe the safeword as a "control" word it can suggest, incorrectly, that it can be used to get one's way. It is a delicate line for a Submissive to figure out the difference between something they just don't like, but are experiencing anyway for other good reasons, versus an event that must stop immediately. My friend Stacey explains it this way, "While I definitely agree that the Submissive has the final control of walking out if things are not to her liking, it's a bit more fuzzy during the actual scene. When I'm with a Dominant, I am surrendered; I don't think through each thing he demands of me to decide whether I'm going to do it or not. After an encounter I might look back on what occurred and decide whether I'm going to stay or go, but while still involved in it, unless my hard limits come up, I am in my partner's complete control." The difference is not between liking the experience or not, but rather being unable, for physical or emotional reasons to continue.

There is also something to be said for experiencing some physical and emotional discomfort in pursuit of a greater goal, perhaps of personal growth, deeper subspace, or greater heights of sensation. If you are feeling that all your experiences are unpleasant, or the relationship as a whole is unpleasant, then you would want to re-evaluate the relationship. After all, if it's not fun, why do it? That includes fun on the intellectual, emotional, and spiritual levels as well as the physical ones. There are so many flavors of both Dominants and Submissives that it's pretty easy to hook up with someone who is not a good match for the long term.

The Submissive having the ultimate control is a great slogan, something which helps make our activities acceptable to the vanilla community, not unlike Safe, Sane & Consensual. SSC is real, but those words are not nearly so clear cut as we'd like vanillas to believe, and in fact are hotly debated within our own community. The usefulness of both these ideas is found in helping vanilla folk understand what we do. It's within our own community that we need to explore the finer points of just who is in control.

* *Green = Great keep going! Yellow = Getting close to Safewording; slow down. Red = Stop!*

Submissives Who Train Their Dominants

Once upon a time, when I had instant messaging active in my e-mail program, guys hit on me pretty much every hour. Presumably being female was enough since God knows they didn't know anything about me as a person. Nowadays with the instant messaging option turned off, I still get a fair number of people coming on to me via e-mail, which is really just as bizarre. Do they not wonder if "Sadie" is really even a woman? Do they not need to know what I do for a living, or where I live, or whether or not I'm a nice person? Presumably not. I suppose many of these people, mostly men, are novices to the BDSM scene or teenagers "trolling." One of the tip-offs is that they so often ask me to "train" them. It's clear they did not put an ounce of thought toward what they might be getting into, or what I as group leader would need out of a partner, or even if I was single!

I receive so many of these messages that I have a form letter for replies. (I'm not kidding). It says something about what I'm looking for in a Dominant, and explains: if they are in bed with me, figuratively speaking, then they are in bed with the BDSM community, with all the joys as well the work and the risks. It may be that no novice is ready to dominate someone who has been the leader of a BDSM group. For one thing, the majority of them have not come out. I, for the most part, have. Most of them are new to having a BDSM community. I'm in the thick of it. But most importantly, they are novices, and as such have neither the skills (how to flog) nor the experience (how long to flog) nor the confidence (when to flog) to be a proper Dominant to someone like me.

For a long time I've been of the opinion that if they had a Dominant mindset, which is mostly confidence, then the skills were secondary. After all, most of it is learned skills, not unlike making a good omelet. I developed this approach partly in hopes it was true, although I hadn't yet substantiated it, but also because it seemed to be a more tactful stance considering the number of novices I interact with on a social basis.

Recently I dated Mal, one of these novices. We had gone out a few times and things were going along well, but he seemed to be having trouble taking control of the situation, of me. No one has ever accused me of being subtle, so I made it clear I was willing to follow any lead he offered. When no lead was forthcoming, I decided maybe Mal just needed a demonstration of what I wanted. I asked his permission to dominate him for five minutes. Being an occasional Dominant myself, I knew exactly what to do. It had nothing to do with toys or skills or practical things. It had everything to do with showing him I was in charge. I did this for a few minutes then invited him to take the helm. Unfortunately, despite my encouragement, he was unable to do so. I repeated this scenario with no less than two other novices with no success.

On thinking this over, I realized I had been quite naive. I thought if Mal saw what to do, his own nature would assert itself. In fact, I think at some level he was scared of me. I guess that's pretty much the bottom line, you just plain can't dominate someone of whom you are afraid.

66

Being a novice is not just about the number of play experiences you've had, or what kind of toys you own, or which books you have read. What differentiates the lions from the kittens is the confidence of having dominated at least one person successfully. Not just any "doormat" Submissive with no self-esteem, but someone who is a whole person. It is a whole different ball of wax to interact with someone who is as strong as you are, physically and mentally.

It may be that this one thing just can't be gotten around. The experience of being in a D/s relationship transforms the players, not just on a superficial level, but on a deeper one. The confidence is not so much about what to do, but in knowing how to take control of another person. There are so few situations in real life where we do anything like this. Even similar experiences or fantasizing or reading about it are simply not it. It's the difference between catering a party and reading recipes. Sure, it's the same adventure in the mind, but the actual doing creates a whole new synaptic connection in the brain. My friend Colby has told me that becoming a Dominant changed not just his sex life, but his whole approach to life. He is more assertive, more patient, and more able to deal with complex situations.

Many novices have suggested I "train" them. I have some friends who tell me they train Dominants, and in fact prefer it because they end up with a custom-made Master. In contrast, in telling someone how, when, and where to spank me, I move into an analytical frame of mind which annihilates the experience of submitting. I also want and need to look up to my Dominant, and it's hard to do this when he's flopping around trying to figure out what to do with me.

Recently I had the experience of playing with Tyler, a high caliber Dominant formally trained in the art of BDSM. I hit on him because I recognized that he could take me to places most

Dominants could not. Tyler didn't have to do anything "to" me to bring out my submissive nature. He simply talked to me, touched me sometimes, and waited for me to respond to the unmistakable fragrance of control. Once, during an early conversation, he took my hand and caressed my wrist. It was probably an erogenous zone thing, and it was probably an opportunity to touch, but it was more than either of those things. Tyler was testing me to see how I would respond when he took control in a small way. And I was testing him too, to see if he could be as easily manipulated as most of the Dominants I know. Tyler didn't need to grope me in the parking lot or have me "demonstrate" how to dominate someone. Most importantly, he didn't allow my flirtation and teasing to invoke his dominant nature. Tyler is in control of himself, and so was in control of me.

Is this because he's a confident, cocky guy? Of course. Is this because he has expensive toys and knows how to use them? A little bit. But are these things enough? No. It is his experience over time which made him "get it," and there may be no way around this for the novice.

That being said, these issues were unimportant when I was starting out in the scene. My first partner Bailey and I didn't know a darn thing between us, so we explored together. There was no pressure on either of us to perform, which worked out quite nicely. Nowadays, I usually recommend this approach to novices.

It may be that I will never be able to interact successfully with a novice, but I do keep the door cracked open in case I was wrong all along. Those "hitting on me" e-mails continue to roll in, but at least now I can explain better how the whole dynamic works, at least for me.

Steamy True Stories of Dominating and Submitting (with a little poetic license)

Dominating

1. One evening in an Indian summer. Sauterelle locked eyes with me. Even as he moved to unzip his pants, his fingers trembled, awkward in an action he must have performed a thousand times. This was his first evening as a Submissive to me. His name means grasshopper, and like a grasshopper he was nervous, as if he might disappear into the silvered moon. But he made it through our dinner of venison and new potatoes, and afterwards asked to display the chastity belt he'd been wearing all week as a gift to me. It was a clear plastic affair, light and practical but ever so tight. His cock strained against the edges, rosy with throbbing. His eyes pleaded and his voice lowered to a softer, more tender timbre. I smiled at his frustration, his need for me to touch him even for just a moment. Even as I reached out, his body shuddered in anticipation.

2. Another night. I grabbed Greghio's hair and pushed him down on my maple table. His face was pressed into the polished wood, but he could still see the array of dildos. Small anal plugs vibrating with a buzz. Medium dongs in pink and black,

with veins and bulbous heads. Gigantic treasures laid down for the fear factor. Greghio mewed, a little in pain and a little in terror. I secured his arms to the table legs, whispering savagely. I stepped between his legs, pulling them too wide, letting him feel the air brush his asshole. This would not be a gentle anal exploration. This would be raping his ass, making him feel like the slut he was. I pressed the dildo against him and he became still with expectation. Waves of need and desperation traveled down his body and into mine, into my legs pressed against his, to my hands holding him down even as I pressed on, invading.

3. Another night. I tied Moby with his arms wide up high and legs spread. I stood behind him, touching, total body contact. As I touched him, tortured him, his pain his desire transferred from his soul to mine, through his hot skin and my teeth on his neck and my fingers dancing over tender places. The sudden intakes of his breath, the shudders, the tears barely withheld. We merged into a circle, a cycle of giving and taking. Pleasure and pain. Submission and dominance. He had made himself completely vulnerable in every way, and I felt each emotion almost as he felt them. We were bound, together.

These are the moments when the dominant side of my nature soared. I knew exactly what each of my Submissives felt, because I had felt it myself. I own him, his body, his soul, his mind, his sexuality. That is the hunger in me, sometimes to feel it in them so I can feel it in myself.

Submitting

1. One evening. Tyler watched me approach. I taunted him, teasing to see if I could invoke his dominance. He put his hand out and stopped me, not with words but with his eyes. He knew better; I knew better. Holding me away from him, he held my forearm and traced a line from my inside of the elbow down to the tip of my middle finger. I couldn't move, drawn in by his power over me. Just a moment, fully clothed, no toys, no anything. Just him staring at me, holding me there firmly in his hold, his dominance.

2. Another evening. Bailey pushed me down over that very same maple table. It was new then, smelling cleanly of pine, custom made at a Vermont furniture store. He lifted my skirt, baring my ass to his hand which crashed upon me, over and over until I didn't think I could take it another second. All I could think of was the pain, of escaping, of not escaping. It burned, and my hands fluttered as I tried to keep from protecting myself from him. My mind became delirious, deranged. I begged him to stop, but he didn't until he had pushed me just a little further, to beyond where I thought I could go. I felt the fabric of his jeans and the hardness of his boots force me open, his hand pulling my hair, holding me still. And then he forced into me, fucking my ass just as I would do years later to another. My first time, a burning helplessness tearing through me even as I knew it was the most right thing. The most right thing.

3. Another winter's evening, too cold for short skirts. Master Jake slouched in my livingroom chair, an eyebrow raised above his sleek silk suit, his arms folded in nonchalance. I walked toward him, twirling my skirt so he could see a whisper of my shaved pussy. He gestured for me to come closer, and I hesitated. What was I thinking

dressing like this so early in our relationship? Surely he would see, he would know how bare I felt, how vulnerable. He told me to spread my legs, and I blushed. I wanted to cry, wanted to shy away. But instead I went forward, and his hand was up and inside me, his fingers finding my clitoris, pulling a moan out of me. He watched me as I stood, unsteady and open, then pulling his hand away in a cool rush of air. He knew. I would give him everything he demanded, and more. All because he showed no fear, no hesitation.

These are the moments when the submissive side of my nature soared. I knew exactly what each of my Dominants felt because I had felt it myself. They owned me, my body, my soul, my mind, and my sexuality. That is another hunger in me, to feel my submission without boundaries.

Part III - Dating in the Scene

Thank heavens I have a sense of humor, because while dating is challenging, dating in the BDSM scene can be one heck of a bear. Here are some stories about my dating life and what I've learned about myself. I think you might find them entertaining, as well as sometimes tender.

The Single Submissive's Lament

Back in the olden days when the BDSM online community consisted of alt.personals.bondage, I had Dominants coming out of my ears and one posted ad could keep me in dinners for a month. Part of this was because I was single, submissive, and female; attributes in high demand. The other part was that I was a relative novice myself and enjoyed the variety of Dominants from the quirky to the bombastic. I admit there were times when I'd rather have been curled up at home with a Robert Parker mystery than listening to some guy spout drivel over porcini tortellini. But generally the dating experience was reasonably entertaining, netting me one or two partners as well as some good friends.

Choosing between all those Dominants was a bit like the restaurant scene here in Burlington. Lots of chain stores like the Olive Garden, but also plenty of family-owned eateries. A Dominant is a Dominant is as a Restaurant is a Restaurant; different but all able to satisfy the basic needs.

One day I started fantasizing about those chicken satay appetizers from Five Spice Café, a wonderful Asian restaurant in downtown Burlington. Even though I still liked Italian,

Vietnamese, and Indian food, they simply could not satisfy my need for chunks of tender chicken draped in peanut sauce. The same thing happened with dating Dominants. After a while my taste became more focused, and I no longer bothered with dating novices, sensation-only players, and anyone outside the Burlington area. It turns out that I'm an impatient and unwilling teacher, relationship oriented, and all too aware few will travel over an hour just for my company. There's just as many players out there these days, but far fewer that are a good match, far harder to order up a good Dominant than a takeout box of chicken satay.

Now that I've gotten a bit known for my writing, I figured it would be much easier to find partners. A prospective Dominant can peruse my website and get the down and dirty on me pretty quick. Not to mention that I know just about everyone in the Northern Vermont community and they all know me. Maybe that celebrity factor is scaring them off or maybe it's the knowledge that I might just write about their sexual proclivities, but I'm dating less now that we have several BDSM groups than when we didn't. The funniest part is that I've scored three Submissives since our community came to be, but only one Dominant, who was not a good match. Then there's the spirituality aspect which I so long to explore, a special interest as unusual as if I were an "enema Dominant" or perhaps a Submissive who was only interested in wallpapering pantries while dressed in a chartreuse dashiki.

A BDSM author friend of mine told me that he gets a lot of "celebrity fuckers" when he travels. I do sometimes get the sense that someone's attracted to me for the glam factor, which is flattering I admit. I have myself suffered from stars in my eyes when meeting well-known scene players for the first time. Somehow I thought they'd be something so much more than I am. But it turns out they they're pretty much like the rest of us, maybe driven by their own particular passion in the BDSM arena, but just as full of crabby moments and questionable character traits. In fact, maybe more negative character traits as the whole glam/celebrity aspect often affects people for the worse. Power corrupts and all that.

Sometimes I wonder if I could just go back to dating vanilla guys, with whom things are so much easier. Well, maybe not easy, but at least overt. We all know the drill: first comes love, then comes marriage, then comes the baby in the.... (fill in the blank). You meet a guy you like, you date. There's no demands that I not wear underwear that evening, or queries about my sex life before the main dish even arrives. No questions about whether I'm "really" submissive. In the vanilla world all that stuff can wait a few months until the sex kicks in.

I imagine my vanilla date picking me up and gazing about while I gather my coat and keys. Mine is a home that clearly belongs to someone with a strong sexual identity. No, there aren't real handcuffs dangling from the wardrobe knobs, but there is the handcuff keychain attached to my spare set of keys. No, there aren't floggers draping the walls, at least downstairs, but there is that red corset embellishing the bedroom door. No, there aren't any "plant hooks" above the dining room table, but the photos of me along the stairwell express an inexplicable sexual aroma. Then there's the copy of The Loving Dominant on the bookshelf, the dominatrix cartoon on the refrigerator, and a pile of unfinished columns by my computer.

Would a pre-date pornsweep manage to disappear all these items? How closely do people look anyway? He might miss the bathroom door and wander into my bedroom where there actually are floggers hanging on the wall, not to mention suspension cuffs and a painting of Isis cradling

Osiris in her arms. His submission to her is unmistakable. What about all these things then?

I see myself explaining to my vanilla date how I spend my time, somehow avoiding the writing, editing, interviewing, and exploring of the BDSM lifestyle. There'd be the untraditional nature of my relationships which would probably give him the wrong idea. I might avoid discussing my experiences in becoming friends with writers, editors, and other interesting scene personalities. That would leave my work, my pets, and a few other hobby oddities. But then something always slips out. I may be able to dissemble at work, but do I want to make that much effort over Asian noodles?

I'm afraid that I will die with dreams still unfulfilled, not "thoroughly used up" as George Bernard Shaw wrote that he wished to be. I dream of a Dominant who doesn't need me to lead him, of a subspace deeper than skin deep, of sex and passion and pain so delirious that I'm lost for a while, far from the construct of my life. Does this even exist, or do I yearn for something impossible, improbable? Am I doomed to live on what I've had so far, interesting, but barely slaking my thirst?

On this summer night, crickets flirt outside my bedroom window, and inside my cats chase each other across the carpet. I am lost, not knowing where and when, or even if he is. If I never find him, would this have been enough, a main dish just barely tasted? Will it be enough hoping that he will, but never actually having felt him claim me? Is it possible to go back in time and be happy with Italian, Vietnamese, and Indian dinners? Or is there only forward to the next level with someone whom I cannot yet imagine? Perhaps he is imagining me even now, and moving ever, perceptibly closer.

Novice on the Precipice

Tonight I went on a date with a novice Dominant whom I met online. The tip-off that Adam was a novice was that he asked me if anything "dangerous" happens at the local munches. I replied that the biggest danger was heartburn from the buffalo wings and occasional boredom from stultifying conversations about pets. But dangerous? Hardly. This would also be a tip off to what would turn out to be a disastrous date.

Adam is a nice enough guy. Mid 30's, pleasant looking, intelligent. I'm those things too, and was dressed in a sporty pink skirt and tank top, hardly D/s fare but then this was Chili's, not Hellfire. As we were walking toward the restaurant I could see he was nervous. "How charming," I thought, "a guy who's actually nervous on a date." Still, he looked more than just a little nervous, more like he was having a panic attack. So we stopped there, mid parking lot, and I asked him to share what was worrying him.

As I looked at his conflicted face, I wondered if somehow I had failed him by not showing up a la Batgirl in a PVC catsuit with a flogger hanging off my belt. Or maybe my lighthearted attitude toward BDSM hadn't matched his serious disposition. Or maybe he hated bottled blondes, or who knows what else about me.

After listening to him stutter half-sentences about being not ready and how it just wasn't right and other things which didn't make much sense, I figured out that no, it wasn't me. It wasn't the restaurant. It was the whole BDSM thing.

I called on my gentle side, the side that was trying to remain calm even as my stomach rumbled and I sensed my dinner receding beyond reach. I reminded him that it was just a bite to eat, that we would talk about our jobs, the weather, and maybe our pets. No kinky sex talk or D/s play in front of the waiter. But it wasn't enough. Adam couldn't walk into the restaurant, much less jaw about life over a mouthful of greasy appetizers. Adam could barely speak.

Somehow, I got this guy on the day, maybe the moment that he was entering the lifestyle. To him, meeting with me represented something, a commitment that he just plain wasn't ready for. I wondered what was the thing that was making him so conflicted. Had he had some terrible sexual experience? Had he been abused? Did he think he might end up abusing me? I imagine that he must have been struggling with fears about sexuality, fears about who he is, what he wants. His fears seemed totally out of proportion to this mild summer evening. I think it wasn't so much about BDSM as it was about him being afraid. Afraid of BDSM, afraid of me, maybe even afraid of life.

With all this, it was hard to imagine Adam as the Dominant that he said he was. Maybe he's only a Dominant in his own mind, which actually isn't all that uncommon. Maybe he's a Pre-Dominant, and won't be ready for full Domliness until he's fully marinated. Finally, I drove home, ranted to a friend, and finished the evening with a load of laundry. This was the first date I'd had that self-destructed in the parking lot. They haven't all been scintillating, but I'd never been cheated entirely. Having things falter this way discombobulated me, although I'm fully aware of how selfish this must sound.

I wonder what he's feeling. Probably guilt-ridden, confused, and scared. Was I any help at all to this terrified novice? I kind of doubt it. Maybe there was nothing I or anyone could have done. I had never met anyone before who was so not-ready to come out. The people who make it to the munches have pretty much passed this phase and are closing in on the racetrack rabbit.

I'd forgotten just how scary the whole BDSM experience can be to a novice. Not all novices of course. Most of them are hungry for experience, peppering me with questions as if I had all the answers. Helping them grow is definitely a job for the teaching souls, not someone like me who is mildly impatient on the best of days. This particular novice needed more than information on how to tie knots and what to wear to the munch. He needed information on how to come to terms with himself. Maybe he has to find himself somewhere within himself before he can reach out. How can we help people who are in that space? Do we even want to?

I don't have many fears anymore; the few I nurtured have been lost in the mists of time. These days I chat with BDSM people all day long. Writers and thinkers. Pro Dommes and editors. Group leaders and ordinary folk like my friend Susan down the block. We gossip about our BDSM lifestyle with the same enthusiasm that we chat about the new Thai restaurant. After ten years it's not hard to talk about my lifestyle, only sometimes hard censoring it when around vanilla people.

The lesson for me is probably that dating novices is a really bad idea. Not having had a date in a month, I had been feeling less discriminating which probably isn't optimal. I did have to remind myself not to take it personally and resist the urge to slap myself for going out with him despite my better judgement. This flopped dinner date was a good reminder that I need someone who is not only experienced in BDSM, but who knows who they are and what they want. No easy thing.

    Still, I'm nothing if not persistent, and so am ready to face down Chili's with yet another Dominant, even if he does turn out to be a Dominant only in his own mind. Either way, as long as there are buffalo wings on the menu, it can't be that dangerous.

Can a Kinky Girl Date a Straight Guy? The Story of my Vacation in Vanillaland

I swore I'd never date a vanilla guy. But then somehow it happened anyway. My friend Makayla and I were at Chili's chowing down on steak fajitas topped with onions and guacamole. I was commenting on how I like men who are men on the outside and women on the inside. Makayla paused mid-chow, looked me straight in the eye and said "I have the man for you."

How could I not believe her? Makayla is of the BDSM persuasion herself, so if her friend Charlie was okay by her, then how bad could he be? Over the next few weeks Charlie and I gossiped on the phone well into the night, and filled each other's e-mail boxes with flirtations. Charlie does indeed have a feminine disposition, and asks intelligent and thoughtful questions like "when you meet people, do you generally like them or generally not like them?" The answer is that I generally like everyone (and they like me) on a superficial level, but I only spend close time with a few. It's a real pleasure to talk with a man who asks me questions and listens to the answers, particularly since I've gotten used to so many blowhards (usually Dominants) talking my ear off without showing the slightest bit of interest in me.

A peek into my photo album will show a series of friends, lovers, all with long hair: black, brown, red, sometimes blond. Usually they have those little glasses which make them look smart, which they are anyway; I love brilliant men. They have a tender disposition, and are able to speak of emotional things with ease. Most interestingly, they are nearly always bisexual, something not nearly as obvious as long hair or little glasses.

Phil (long black hair and little glasses) was the first. When he "confessed" he was bisexual, I laughed and said I already knew. He was shocked! Similar to "gay-dar," the way gays recognize each other ("gay" plus "radar"), I have "bi-dar." There's more to chemistry than charm, wit, and hairspray.

So here I was with Charlie, another guy who fit the framework pretty well. Well maybe he did not have the long hair and little glasses, but as my sister says, hair grows and eyesight can go to hell. Would it work with a vanilla guy? Of all the couples I know in the BDSM community, only one has a truly vanilla partner, and I have yet to pin them down and get them to explain how they make it work. Charlie and I discussed some of relationship options where couples often keep sex for each other, but do BDSM play with other people. Would something like this work for a guy who was a pretty traditional sort, the sort who was married for ten years and believed in sticking by your woman no matter what? Hard for me to imagine though he seemed willing enough.

Charlie said he found the BDSM lifestyle kind of interesting, if a little scary. He said he'd give it a try, dip his toes in. His attitude reminds me of years ago when I asked my partner Garrett to wear his leather chaps to the bedroom. The feel and smell of the leather turned me on something fierce, but the truth is, Garret was pretty vanilla and no amount of dressing up could make a Dominant out of him. I wonder if any amount of toe-dipping could make Charlie into a Dominant either. Probably not.

On the other hand, my friends Gary and Rebecca were mostly vanilla when they met, and today he is a contributing editor to Prometheus Magazine (one of the preeminent BDSM rags) and she's the moderator of Leatherchurch (for BDSM souls exploring the spiritual side of things). Were they attracted to each other by some unspoken, unconscious thing just as I am naturally drawn to gentle and tender men? Surely they could not have guessed that years later they'd be knee-deep in BDSM. Was that luck or something deeper?

Maybe because I was enjoying talking to Charlie so much, I'd forgotten how exotic we BDSM folk appear to vanilla people, to him. My friend Queen Maureen describes it this way, "One thing I like about the BDSM community is the way relationships can have so many different levels. In the vanilla world, you either are involved with someone, or you are not. In the BDSM world, I can have multiple submissives, all at different points in the relationship. I can date, play, be friends, whatever and it is what it is. I can live with one submissive, date someone vanilla, play with friends, and it is okay."

Maureen goes on to describe how a friend of hers "complained about a new girlfriend and how she wants commitment and he isn't ready. Their rules are so black and white, they broke up." Turns out the rules for Charlie are black and white in the same way. It was one thing for him to consider dating someone like me, but he needed to know what our relationship would or could be: "casual dating" or "friendship with privileges" or what exactly? I don't know exactly what I told him; I'm pretty fluid about these things. I guess that was a bit too loosey goosey for Charlie or any typical red-blooded American guy.

Worse, Charlie felt I considered sex a "recreational activity." His comments may be a reflection of my lighthearted attitude toward sex, or my willingness to explore alternative relationships. Since I have been celibate for months, it doesn't make a lot of sense to me. If I'm going to do sex recreationally, I should at least be getting some. Either way, to Charlie my way of living wasn't as serious as his, and so he went his way and I went mine.

What we are doing, this open approach of relationships, is more than just a little different from the vanilla norm. It's a whole different enchilada, one which is scary and maybe even a bit sleazy to vanilla people in general, and Charlie in particular. Our sexualized community may be a perfect fit for my bawdy girl style, but I'm thinking that this time, I really swear I won't date vanilla again!

Going on a Dating Sabbatical, and the One who Slipped in Under the Wire

If you've been reading along with me on my Single Submissive series, you know my last two dating adventures were more like dating debacles. It's not so much that there's something wrong with the guys I dated, rather that I'm clearly rummaging in the wrong sale bin. In response to a bit of low-key whining on the subject, my friend Susan suggested I go on a "dating sabbatical." She had been on a sabbatical from refined sugar and thought the experience was giving her some perspective. I agreed, and declaring myself a non-dating Submissive, promptly removed the "dating resume" from my website. I may not be getting any more now, but calling it a dating sabbatical sounds more glamorous.

During my decision-making process, I'd been swapping pert e-mail with a Dominant who'd slipped in under the wire. He'd located me through one of those singles boards a day before I pulled the ad. I wondered, what's a girl to do? Again Susan came to the rescue, advising me to follow through with Trevor and see where it might lead. "After all," she said, "the idea of a sabbatical is to get perspective, not to cling to an artificial construct."

A week later I'm still officially not dating, but Trevor and I have been heating up the wires with lively conversation. He has a creative turn of mind as well as eight years experience as a Dominant. According to his photos he is a pretty good looking guy, and likes a gal with fabulous boobs; so we're all set there. I have the sense he could control me; a pleasant, if unusual sensation. He describes himself as on the "fringe" of the scene, in contrast to my being cleavage deep. Trevor is confident we will make a good match, but I remain the cautious optimist. I've had plenty of first dates where the guy turned out to have engaged in false advertising. One date sent (what turned out to be) a ten year old photograph; sharp and smart in his Canadian mountie uniform. In person he was out of shape, unemployed, and wearing a T-shirt decorated with food stains. His mountie days were long gone as were the chances of us going on a second date. You bet I'm cautious; no butterflied prawns entre makes up for chemistry gone awry.

Trevor is not alone in equating the e-mail/phone experience to being with someone in person. Ludicrous, I say. When you are talking on the phone with someone you are in essence telling them the story of your life, an edited version with highlights on the dramatic and entertaining parts; not unlike my columns. Nothing wrong with this, but it is not real life.

In person you can observe the subtleties of your date's personality: how they deal with bad drivers, whether or not they can take out the trash without being reminded, and if their checking account is balanced. Only in person can you observe how he steamrolls people who disagree with them, or how he has become so obsessed with BDSM that he has forgotten how to be anything else, or how his emotional issues prevent him from keeping a job. These are not figmental Dominants of my imagination, rather very real men, although fortunately not ones I've been involved with. Each is intelligent and charming online where storytelling is easy, yet unable to maintain offline.

Sadly, I can't tell Trevor that he's the right Dominant for me, or even the Dominant for right now. I enjoy talking with him on the phone, allow him to arouse me aurally, but commit to nothing. Bucking the trend of self-disclosure I refrain from sharing too intimate details of my personal life until we know each other better. That's okay though, because I'm really not dating you know, I'm on a sabbatical.

Part IV - Diary Of A Journalist Submissive: My Adventures In Formal Training

This is a series exploring my formal training by Master Dex at House Mermaid in "Mermaid Falls," New York (near Albany). It was written as events actually unfolded. It's helpful to read this series in order, but not absolutely necessary.

Exploring the Possibility of Formal Training as a Submissive

This all might have started last September, when for the first time I asked a Dominant to train me in a formal manner. The negotiation was a dismal failure, not because of the content of what we were negotiating, but because our communication styles hailed from different planets. So one might wonder why, just six months later, am I making another attempt?

This week, a confluence of other events got my butt in gear. The main one is that a BDSM publisher, expressed interest in publishing a book of my writing. My manuscript was not long enough, and so I agreed to write another 25,000 words in the next three months. What on earth would I write about? It's true enough that I can write up a storm, but then something as specialized as BDSM seems to need a little push. I decided to pursue some formal training as a Submissive and so bushwhack some of the 25,000 word mountain while having a bit of fun.

My first step was to write a little proposal to my friend Dex, a Master who owns House Mermaid. He had actually communicated with me some time ago, but I responded to him with the usual brush off, as I do with the majority of e-mail "hits" I receive. He and his partner barbie live some three hours away, which isn't conducive to my lifestyle. On the other hand, Dex isn't just playing around with BDSM, he lives it. He's the kind of person I need to guide me to the next level.

So when I spent time with him at a local munch, I was initially attracted to the fact that he had clearly made a lifestyle choice. I am also no fool, and I checked around to see if Dex is the person he purports to be. The word was that he had a good reputation, and also that there were some politics involved. Politics I know about; there are politics in my BDSM life too.

What I wanted was someone who had the confidence and competence to dominate me. It had to be someone who knew himself, and was emotionally grounded. In a world with thousands of novice Dominants rattling around, these qualities are difficult to find. While I'm entertained by Dex's investment in his dungeon and toy collection, they are not just window dressing, but an indicator of his commitment to the lifestyle.

I suggested to Dex that he take me on in a training capacity with two goals: to teach me some elements of a formal and traditional style, as well as allow me to write about the experience as it unfolded. He explained that he uses a combination of Old Guard, Eastern, and European practices in his approach, making his style unique and not easily comparable to other BDSM houses. My feeling about this is, I don't really care in which style I am trained. My interest is in the experience of being trained itself, not in the mechanics. I know that when I move on to a more permanent Master, many of the things I learned will have to be re-learned. That's not my concern, however. What I want to understand is what it is to be trained, and what training is.

My experience so far with Masters has been with what could be called "Weekend Warriors." These are masters who may vary from novices to experienced players, but none of them are lifestyle players. I think of "lifestyle players" as people who have made a greater commitment to BDSM, a commitment which is reflected in their time invested, hobbies, friends, and community. With Weekend Warriors, we'd get together with them for an evening for dinner and a few hours of play. While we'd certainly have fun, and over time explore many of the BDSM flavors, there was a playful quality to our interactions. There was no training of any sort, and no interest in learning any kinds of formal protocol. This is not to say that this is true for all weekend players, of course, only the ones with whom I've been involved.

So, while I feel I have experienced a wide variety of BDSM play, I have not felt what it is to submit on a deeper level, not just for those few hours and for some play of one sort or another, but as a whole person. I'm not sure how I'd react to a situation like this, but I certainly am very interested in exploring it, both as a Submissive and as a writer.

For the record, I have never received training of any sort. So if the truth be told, I haven't the faintest idea of what Dex's training will entail. We have planned some time to go over this in detail as well.

That's about where things stand at the moment. As I complete negotiations with Dex and hopefully move into a training situation, I'll continue to write about my experiences. My hope is that both I and my readers learn something about this kind of BDSM through my experiences.

Why This?

A few people who like me less than I'd prefer, have accused me of being a BDSM weekend warrior. They're right. I may spend a lot of time writing about the dynamics of D/s, but my real life revolves not around play, but around the usual suspects: work, home, and family. In the hierarchy of some people in our community, my approach is just too darn provincial. They may be right about the label, too, but then Dorothy and I have always known that everything we need is in our own back yards.

I always thought of "lifestyle" folk as the ones living it up in the big cities: Boston, Atlanta, and New York City. Every night a different club, where naked strangers are lashed to giant wheels, and twirled upside-down to the wind accompaniment of floggers, whips, and crops. I hear about BDSM houses and dungeons where people live 24/7. In my fevered imagination, they wear spiked collars all day long, scrub kitchen floors with ratty toothbrushes, and give foot massages with their tongues. All this while muttering mantras of ownership. I hear about friends who spend every weekend traveling to one play party or another, ratcheting up yet another scene on their belt. On to the next Jeeves; another day, another flogging!

Are any of these images real? Who knows. They resonate because they are so far from my real life experience as to assume a cartoonlike coloring. I don't do any of these things, fevered imaginings or not, and probably never will. Even if I liked to travel, which I don't, I'm not interested in casual play. Nor do I enjoy big groups or noisy clubs. Despite my reputation, I'm a writer first, and we writers are a quiet, contemplative lot.

BDSM is my sexual orientation, not who I am or how I live my life. It is not who I am as a human being, and not even how I choose to spend most of my time. I am myself first and a Submissive second.

Still, I wonder sometimes what is hidden behind curtain number three. Sure, I've had my share of experiences. Being Submissive. Being Dominant. Being in between. I've tried most of the things that piqued my interest, met a variety of players from the banal to the spicy, have collected a few choice toys. At the moment I'm waiting for another love, the kind which will take my D/s explorations deeper into the soulful space.

But what of the meantime? How long can a lustful girl like myself go on without gratification? It's been almost a year since I decided to no longer play casually. I did weaken for a single one-night stand. I have entertained myself in the last few months with a novice Dominant, but neither could ease the yearnings of my submissive soul, which wants, which needs release.

I began to wonder if herein was the space where I might explore something completely new and different. A formal training seems so foreign to me, it might change some of my ideas about who I am. Formal training seems so alien to my informal approach to BDSM, and I wonder why even bother when the Dominants of my experience could care less? They never truly wanted to control me, my whole sexuality for more than a few hours at a time, and even so I knew deep down that there were no real punishments. There was never a time where they really pushed me, beyond what I thought I could take or wanted to take. No matter what I was experiencing, we both knew it would be over in a few hours and we'd be on the phone ordering pizza with extra cheese and sun dried tomatoes.

What if I were to commit to real training as a Submissive? What if things didn't have an assumed end when we both got winded and needed a bite to eat? What would it be like to have someone control me in deeper ways, for longer, with a commitment to obeying even when it was not something I actually wanted to do? What would it be like to be punished for real, not the "oh you're so bad I'm going to punish you" kind of punishment, but the real thing, punishment until I wept. What would it be like to suffer just because he wanted me to? Would I struggle against it with every fiber of my independent soul? Or would those parts of me drift off in a puff of breeze, leaving me settled and safe in his arms?

I want to know these things. I want to feel the real turn-over of my self, when I suffer not because I am a masochist, but because suffering for him will take me to the next level. I want to feel that "lift: when my own wants and needs and demands recede into the background; when submission is not just for the evening, but for the weekend, for the week, for all of me.

This is the why, of why I'm exploring a relationship with Dex. It's not for his intellectual mind or his experience with one toy or another. It's not his BDSM house or that he's not intimidated by me or my personae. It's because I think, I hope, that he can say "no" to me in a way that few can. I think he might take my hand and lead me down long corridors, deep into the dark places of my mind, deep into the mysterious places I haven't seen for sure, but which I know are there. Deep into the places where only the soul knows.

The First Weekend

Despite the broken down factories littering the road into the little town of Mermaid Falls, the citizens clearly still believe in the power of artistic expression. On one corner, a house painted entirely in whimsy, with bright faces of purple and green laughing at the neighborhood. On the next block, a brick building with a farm scene painted thirty feet high and even wider. A little further, a home hidden behind a hundred stuffed and fully dressed bunnies hanging out in the yard, drinking tea and presumably chatting about the upcoming Easter holiday.

Dex and barbie's home is cared for with the same level of attention. A 100 year-old Victorian of grey with pink trim. Tall ceilings and antique wallpaper. Shining wood floors and thousands of square feet between the two floors of living space, full upper dungeon, and a basement which will one day be a finished lower dungeon. It's a good thing Dex and barbie found this house in such fine condition, because it's clear they've spent an inordinate amount of time, love and money turning it into more than just a house, into House Mermaid.

As if the house itself weren't enough, Dex is fortunate to have extensive woodworking skills, as well as a few carpenter friends. The result is a fully finished attic dungeon with soaring ceilings edged with colored lights. Three cages, three Saint Andrew's crosses, bondage and waxing beds, stocks and too many other props to mention. The room is warm with portable heaters and dramatic lighting, and practical with handy storage cabinets of first aid and safety materials.

Could there be more? There is, and I found it in Dex and barbie's bedroom which hosts not only his custom-made bondage bed, but a toy collection which outshines anything I have ever witnessed. A wall of floggers, not the $50 kind I have in my own modest collection, but the $200+ kind from the big names. A rack of whips of every color, style, and make, the kind of top-quality whips a master of this tool would have. Cuffs, crops, paddles, feathers, and more.

Yes, I was impressed with the breadth and depth of Dex's love of BDSM accoutrements, but then, most of the guys I know collect BDSM toys; it's almost a genetic predisposition. If his stuff had been all there was, I would not have bothered with him, not to mention I hardly need his toys as I have my own toy bag. House Mermaid is only partly about the paraphernalia, however. More important to Dex and barbie is their extended family of affiliated members to the house. Four couples in all make a cohesive family, one who is there in good times of winning ice hockey games and bad times of hospital visits. A family who visited for dinner and shared conversation with me over tender roasted chicken and diane's famous ambrosia for dessert. A family who helps produce the monthly play parties, as well as their collaring ceremonies, and other private events.

You might wonder then where would I fit into all this? What I do know is that Dex is everything he appears. A man who commits himself with the same dedication to choosing just the right collar for me as he does in choosing the structure of his lower dungeon. He takes everything seriously, and every item, every person in his life is there and close to his heart. There are few things which are casual with him. When I observed him doing a scene with barbie, his attention and focus were unmistakable. His love and attention for her is not superficial, but deep down. He encourages her financial independence so she will not become so dependant on him and be unable to function on her own. I found this fascinating, because it would be so much easier for a control-freak type to control everything indiscriminately. Dex chooses to give her independence, meaning that she stays because she chooses to, not because she can't function otherwise. If nothing else, this act told me more about Dex than the hundreds of toys lined up on his bedroom walls.

But Dex doesn't come to me as a single unit. He has built this house, this family out of a need for loved ones nearby. I admire his dedication and the obvious affection his family members have for him and each other. My situation is quite different, with little family and few responsibilities outside of my own muse. On the good side, the thought of being welcomed into a family like this is very attractive. Who wouldn't want an instant community? On the other side, each person you add into the mix changes things. And God knows I am no shy flower. I'm more likely to pop up with a few controversial topics during the post-ambrosia conversation. Will they want a person like me around? I don't know, and perhaps that will be the crux of things down the line.

When I first started negotiating with Dex, I thought of the situation as a training thing primarily between him and me, with deference to barbie as alpha Submissive. I didn't quite realize that House Mermaid is not just a house, not just a giant collection of toys, not just an idea. In fact, House Mermaid is a fully realized vision of a cohesive lifestyle, a confluence of people, location, and events. Is there space for another person in this meeting place? I wonder.

The last morning, we sat around the breakfast table munching on perfectly crisp bacon which Dex had cooked up long before any of us had awakened. We scrutinized the paperwork; the checklists, the health questions, and the actual contract of submission. Dex is not a bossy Dominant and has negotiated with me every step of the way. He takes my concerns seriously and responds thoughtfully. We ended the weekend with a flurry of hugs, but nothing signed. On the next visit we will perhaps venture into the contract signing, complete with new collar, and a whisperings of things to come. The mystery of my journey has yet to begin, but we've done a very good job of building the foundation.

Dex And Me

    I felt the collar click at the back of my neck, Dex's arms heavy on my shoulders, his breath warm in my ear. Its antique silver closure connects a black cord and a small silver ring. Nothing big and dramatic, but more than I had ever committed to before. Over this, Dex laid a silver necklace with intertwined mermaids, singing, swimming at the bottom, a symbol of my affiliation to House Mermaid. I hugged Dex and barbie who both smiled at me, and so I was collared for the first time.
    We strode inside to the Vermont munch. This was the first time I had ever attended a public function with a Dominant. I'd attended several with my own Submissives, but of course that's a different ball of wax. I felt that whatever Dominant I brought to the public arena must be equal to me, not a novice who was not out enough, or up to the challenge of laughing in the face of speculation. There was the competition aspect as I was in a leadership role, a dominant role.
    I am not unaware of the public and hierarchical aspects of our relationship. I didn't choose Dex for political reasons, but I am aware of the unique place he has in the Albany BDSM community. In some ways, Dex has taken the path less traveled in a community as rife with politics

as anywhere else. After all, power struggles are always a factor, and ten times worse when you have a community of people who groove on the power exchange. I've always been one to bet on the dark horse.

Maybe there is a part of me that jives on being a bit controversial. I'm not known for being a team player, even in my own community, particularly in my own community. I am an artist, an auteur with a vision, which broadly translates to Don't Get In My Way. I know my personae and my writing bring a certain cachet to Dex and House Mermaid. Of course for me to affiliate with a house, I want it to reflect my vision as well. House Mermaid reflects that vision in ways which may not be obvious on the surface, but which are nevertheless true.

Dex started my formal training this weekend. During most of the munch, I was "tethered" to him by the six foot rule, which I failed only once while lost in passionate conversation with Sir Ron and Mayafire, the leaders of APeX (shop talk gets me every time). The next day he started training me to say "Sir" when I spoke to him. This has been difficult for me, particularly in front of fellow players. Mostly I feel a little ridiculous, but at times it feels pleasant and respectful to say it. There are other things like dropping my eyes for a moment when I meet a Dominant. And more. At the moment, I do what he asks to please him, although for the most part these actions have no real meaning for me. He has explained to me the philosophy of respect and submission that his rules reflect, and I expect my understanding will become deeper with time.

In our first official scene together, I lay on the waxing table which has a marble insert. The idea is to have one side cool while the other side is heated by the paraffin wax. The room, set off from the upper dungeon, has dark walls and glow-in-the dark stars lit by black light for a spectacular effect. For this first time, Dex was inordinately careful with me, checking in with me constantly, attending me with affection and focus. Of all the toys which floated across me, tickled and drifted and caressed, the one that did me the most was the Vampire Gloves. They are leather gloves with little sharp studs built in, and when pressed suddenly into my nipples they nearly brought me off the table. He wanted to know if I was turned on, and indeed I was, although I didn't articulate it very well. The cold metal burned through my nipples and drove directly downward. Yes I was hot, but perhaps too perplexed and distracted by this, our first scene, to respond.

Of course I think Dex was too kind, too gentle with me. I need much more. I also know he is a responsible Dominant and he's just doing his job, as they say. I don't know if I was in subspace so much as just in an intensively sensual place. Afterward I slumped over the couch to stare at the news, unable to take in a single word; I suppose I must have gone somewhere, somehow.

This feeling of being owned is nearly unfamiliar. Although I've been with plenty of Dominants, they were not the "owning" sort. I like the feeling of quiet safety I have with Dex. My friend Kaitlyn described Dex's energy as a positive force, and I agree. Dex is stable and dependable – a lot like me actually – and a lot unlike the artsy lost souls I've been dating recently. He is a doer, always active: cooking, creating, connecting. He is an "easy" Master in that he feels free to do dishes, and act in ways which may on the surface not appear to be "Dominant." He is protective toward me and touches me periodically to reorient me to his direction. His caress is warm, and I feel a quiet safety when I'm with him. Not safe as in I was ever at risk, but grounded on a deeper level, one which is difficult to articulate.

Still I don't want to be a Pollyanna about Dex, who is as human as the rest of us. Dex has been in a three year 24/7 relationship with a very particular kind of Submissive, the kind barbie is.

He is learning how to negotiate a relationship with someone like me, a very particular kind of someone who is very different than barbie. This is a new experience for him, and it shows in how he is learning to ask me questions and listen to the answers. He knows barbie so well that with her, few questions are needed. I can see it's a bit of a struggle for him, as he's not an emotionally oriented person. When I venture into the emotional realms, he tends to drift off a bit, which he tells me is something of a reaction to a difficult childhood.

Although I obviously don't need protection, Dex provides it anyway. There is part of me which finds it bizarre, and another which finds it pleasant. For example, when we were at the munch, Dex came with me to the bathroom. He told me he does this because he wants to protect his Submissives from the sharks who sometimes attend BDSM functions. I appreciate his philosophy and don't make a fuss, although anyone who knows me could more likely imagine me ka-powing some guy in the kisser for giving me a hard time.

What is more challenging for me to resolve is that Dex's approach could perpetuate a culture of fear. Fear that bad Dominants are out there waiting to hurt us Submissives. Fear that Submissives won't be able to protect themselves and so will be hurt in some way. People might say that I haven't ever felt at risk because I'm a confident woman and all, but it's hard to say. In any case, I believe that most of our experiences are not objective realities, but rather perceptions that we have created for ourselves. I don't believe in Truth (with a capital T).

In a similar way, my friend Ryan believes his male friends betray him, and sure enough they do, hearing him tell it. Yet, my friends never betray me. Is it because I have chosen different kinds of friends, or is it that the word, the concept of "betrayal," is not in my lexicon? It's such a loaded term, dramatic. Events happen in my life as they do in his, but he sees them as a betrayal while I see them as unpleasant experiences. Sometimes of course I am hurt, but I know it's ultimately about them, not about me.

Despite our differences in approach, I think Dex and I make a good team. Choosing him reflects my increasing ability to make good choices when it comes to BDSM partners, which is a good thing for me. I like the things I'm learning both from him personally, and from my experiences at House Mermaid.

I also like the changes which are happening inside me. There is a certain freedom that comes with the collar, although I can see how it might appear to be the opposite. On the surface I no longer have to put energy into looking for a partner, or getting to know Dominants who for the most part are not up to the job. It saves me time and energy. My submissive nature has not been attended to in a very long while. So on a deeper level, being cared for frees me from unfulfilled needs. I can't say exactly what I can do now which I couldn't do before, only that there is something inside me which has relaxed just a little bit. It may have nothing to do with the actual collar around my neck, but then it just might.

My Polysomething Relationships

Years ago, well before my BDSM coming out, a couple I knew described their polyamorous relationship and invited me to join them. I was so flummoxed that my mouth continued to gape even as I stumbled out the door, never to speak with them again. Thinking on things now, I wonder why it pushed such buttons in me. After all, I've had open relationships since my high school days, when my very first lover kissed my cherry. Is the step to polyamory such a big one?

I have an idea this all started when I was on a break from college classes, and my mother told me that she and my dad had engaged in an open relationship. She explained that they loved each other, but wanted to explore other avenues. They had done a good job of hiding it because we kids never had a clue. The revelation weirded me out a bit but somehow the idea must have sprouted in my unconscious because a few months later my partner Garrett and I made the same decision.

Garrett and I loved each other, but after four years together we needed some spice. So, we developed groundrules such as safe sex and no messing about in our homespace. We agreed on total honesty and a "no drama" policy. We started out keeping the episodes private from each other, but we soon found that sharing the juicy parts made a hot little addition to our sex life. In the three years following, I never felt jealousy or anger. I knew Garrett loved me, and so I also knew there was nothing to fear. This, however, isn't polyamory technically speaking. If either of us had fallen in love with someone else, we would have separated; that was the deal. As a sometime Dominant I am far more proprietarial about my Submissives, but don't mind sharing them as long as it's on my terms.

Some say if you let your partner go gallivanting around, you can't complain if they fall in love with someone else. They claim you opened the door, and too bad if you don't like the consequences. I have a problem with this both philosophically and practically. The main thing is that I loved and trusted Garrett. I can not, and will not, live in fear that he might fall in love with someone else. If it's going to happen, it's going to happen and having sex with other people is not going to, in itself, create love where love was not. In putting sex, love, and boundaries out in the open, the intrigue disappears, and the act loses its power to hurt. Sex is not the same as love, and you can't create love out of sex any more than you can create love out of wishful thinking. When it's all on the table, your relationship is one of choice, not of victimization.

All of my relationships have been nontraditional in one way or another. Maybe it's because I have such a craving for offbeat tastes, but not a single one has been strictly monogamous in the way most Americans define it. Some were love relationships like the one with Garrett where we had agreements on what and when and how we could get some on the side. Others were more casual lovers, both D/s and vanilla, to whom I had no commitment, even though I may have been with them for years. Several were one or a few night stands.

I don't know what this all makes me, not polyamorous probably, but polysomething.

People throw around the polyamorous word a lot, and it encompasses a lot of things. When you're talking about sharing love with multiple adult partners, it seems to be much harder to maintain than sharing only sexual or D/s play. Getting along with one person is a fair bit of work on the emotional and spiritual scales. Getting along with two is an exponential increase, the kind which results in so much emotional processing that I want to rip my pubic hair out. Probably not a good choice for me, but then you never know.

One of the issues I've struggled with is that in our culture, monogamy is assumed to be the optimal goal. If you choose alternative lifestyle relationships as I have, there's an underlying assumption that somehow you either weren't worthy of having someone commit to you fully or you have some kind of commitment problem yourself. There's also a misconception that in an open relationship you are swinging with every penis flapping in your breeze. How ridiculous.

I've thought a lot about these things, mostly because it irritates me so to be judged. Our family upbringing offered far more options than marrying and banging out a few kids, neither of which I have done. My parents might not have told their children about their open relationship until we were adults, but their underlying beliefs in our ability to choose the paths of our lives made the difference between living my life my way and being trapped in society's expectations of women. Having poly relationships, broadly speaking, does not seem at all odd to me; it's been completely normalized in my mind. The only time I notice how unusual it is happens when I tell a vanilla friend about it. Most of them raise a few eyebrows, and I didn't even get to the D/s part yet...

Do I have a commitment problem then? I don't think so. When I have been in love, I committed easily. Otherwise I haven't. I have always valued my independence, perhaps so much it often eclipsed the need for a relationship. Is this a choice or something else? I believe it's the former because I feel that God has been with me every step of the way. I am no victim.

What then is it that Dex, barbie, and I have? Yes, Dex loves barbie. He likes me, and I think she likes me too. At the moment we're still independent organisms, toddling along side by side, interacting when it's convenient. I don't know if somewhere down the line we will develop something deeper. Certainly it seems natural for feelings of some sort to develop under the aegis of such intimate contact.

I wonder how barbie feels about me. I imagine she feels the uncertainty any Submissive would feel when things change. She will presumably have a little less time with Dex for the hours he spends with me. After three years there must be long periods where they're living side by side, and I could presumably slip in without barely making a ripple. But maybe this is ingenuous. I won't call this polyamorous since that isn't what we are doing, but it is nevertheless a non-traditional arrangement with some of the same complexities.

I have told barbie that she has nothing to fear from me, but such assurances may be meaningless. For who could promise that I won't fall in love with Dex, or somehow, some way, provide him with something that she doesn't. In fact, by definition I already provide him with something she doesn't, if only because we are so different. What is it like for her, a gentle quiet spirit to have me around, colorful, outspoken, unrestrained? I don't know. I've never been in her position, and probably can't even imagine it. I don't see this as a bad thing. Each of us is on a path, not fate, but one that we have mostly chosen. Whatever changes I bring to their relationship are the ones which are right not only for me, but also for them by virtue of them having made their own choices. I have faith in the process. I don't know if they live by the same belief system. I imagine it might be hard for her, yet I don't imagine I can do this work for her. She has to process it out herself.

I can see how my presence affects others, affects Dex and barbie. On the one hand, there's the Star Trek Prime Directive: to leave things as I found them. I did leave their kitchen as I found it, but in a relationship that is impossible. We are all changed by the presence of another. I came into this relationship with Dex and barbie with no hidden agenda, and I don't think they had one either. No drama, no artifice. I know people sometimes come into poly relationships not knowing themselves well enough to know what they want, and things then deteriorate into a big mess. In a situation like this, you really need to know who you are and what you want, because if you don't, no amount of well-intentioned communication can glue together the cracked Humpty Dumpty of trust.

These days I barely blink an eye when someone suggests a new relationship flavor, and I'm unlikely to run out of the room regardless of the oddness of the offer. I have come to terms with the pattern of my life and the fact that it's not conforming with much in the vanilla world. It does seem very welcome in the BDSM world, and that's the one where I belong.

Cupid, Collars, and Commitment

During their "first dance" after the collaring ceremony, Madam Saki leaned in close toward Cole her Submissive and whispered "I love you." I captured the moment on digital film, just as it captured my imagination. Does she really love him? Is it the heart-shaped boxes of chocolates and walks on the beach kind of love? Or does D/s eros take on a different flavor, tangy with a darker juice?

Of course, they weren't doing the waltz kind of dancing either, but rather his first public scene, attended by the extended family at House Mermaid. There is a different way of things in D/s relationships. I have completed the preliminary negotiations with Dex, and so we have also completed what in the vanilla world might be the "dating" phase. We checked each other out, explored our chemistry, got references, and tested the waters successfully on a few divisive issues.

Now I wear a collar of consideration, which might be like "going steady." We have made a commitment, even if a short one, to exploring together, and the collar tells our respective communities: "hands off."

Madam Saki has accepted Cole's petition for the next step, the training collar, which might be analogous to a marriage. For the next six months, they will be in the honeymoon period of a new relationship. She tells me their eroticism is not the glossy fluffed hair sexuality of porn magazines, but about control, about serving her needs, about sensuality. I see her sensuality in the way she draws close to him in a scene, whispers softly, intimately. He smiles back, vulnerable.

When the hormones have cooled, as they often do, the ownership collar will be the commitment for the long term, a deeper affection than could ever be present or even imaginable after my few months with Dex, or after Cole's few months with Madam Saki. This is what Dex and barbie have, different than vanilla love, more than just play.

We signed our contracts together over breakfast, with witnesses gazing down on us with a benevolent look in their eyes. In some ways, this commitment is more than I've made to any man in years. My two relationships since Moby were transition ones, designed to get me through my grief and out the other side intact, or at least functioning. But this commitment is in alignment with my shift from casual love, casual play, casual relationships to something more. Not so sure what that more is, but I'm working on it.

Not everyone takes that approach, however. There is a very real appeal to being a couple in the scene, even more than the general cultural pressure to pair up. For some who are interested in the hierarchies of things, couples can be seen as more stable, as higher in the hierarchy. Of course, I'd disagree with that particular worldview, as I tend to take the "economics" approach, with women like myself being more in demand and so being of higher "value." The bottom line of course, is that these are all artificial constructs. Each of us is valuable exactly to the degree which we believe ourselves to be. Within the community though, experience counts, and people like Dex with something to offer besides his good looks and charm are in demand.

There is a joy in owning someone. Looky here! Look what I snagged on my line. This pretty or sexy or servile person will do my bidding; suffer for me, clean for me, pleasure me on my whim. There is a joy in being owned as well. This person makes me more valuable; I am owned by someone of experience and stature. Yes this does all sound pretty crass, maybe even juvenile. But crass or not, it's also sometimes true. I accept it and at the same time want to go beyond it. I want to explore deeper, both on a personal level and a cultural level.

Madam Saki's collaring ceremony is only the second collaring I've ever attended. The first one I witnessed was relatively casual, although touching in its simplicity. This one was more formal, just a training collar, but a commitment still taken seriously. Madame Saki dressed in red silk with a layer of black lace, a rose curved into her breast. Her Submissive, Cole, showed off his body, tall and lithe in a leather harness. He also dressed in a shy smile, which created adorable dimples. He's so very young, I thought, and he is, just 21. Already he knows his path. Does he know how lucky he is to have found someone like Madam Saki, with her wicked sense of humor? She reaches out to me, a stranger, and connects with an undeniable warmth.

They exchanged roses and vows, and we stood in a circle, warmed by the light of leather-scented candles and a riot of flowers. We blessed their union as they bless our community.

Afterward, during their First Dance in the attic dungeon, Cole was still shy, even as he blushed, showing the proper forms she'd taught him. Loose and limber as he rested fully into the floor holding his kowtow position. He was beautiful in his devotion, beautiful beyond his sweet boy toy look.

So then what is this relationship? Madam Saki tells me it's not sex, not eros, not romantic love. She says it is more of the philos flavor of love, brotherly love (which of course is why Philadelphia, the city of brotherly love is so named). No, not about sex, but about a caretaking and teaching relationship. She has other Submissives, and bottoms herself sometimes, sometimes with Dex or another Dominant, sometimes not. Sometimes with love, sometimes not. Always with passion, and a massive streak of exhibitionism.

Other couples are together in other ways. Dex tells me he loved barbie when she moved in as a 24/7 Submissive, but in retrospect it was only a fashion of love, lighthearted and light. It was only after he'd lived with her for a few months that they fell in love deeply, eclipsing the experiences he'd had with his two former wives.

Lady Midnite and samri, another couple and affiliate of the house, tell me their connection was love and lust at first sight, falling into each other's arms the very night they met. An unlikely couple she says, because she always went for the tall military types, but then cupid's flogger is nothing if not something to be reckoned with. The affection between them is unmistakable, despite that samri is more my type than hers, a gentle, feminine soul with an artistic temperament. He is the house pet, cheerful in his role as the smart-assed masochist, and modest in his ability to both self-bind and self-suspend himself from the equipment that indeed, he and Dex built. Lady Midnite is his opposite, with a raucous laugh and an easy manner. I think she probably didn't trust me right off, but she seems to have softened toward me some. She has allowed me to see not only her bitchy mistress self, but also her deep affection for samri.

In arranged marriages couples learn to love each other, or presumably sometimes they don't. In interviews with women from the Middle East, many of these women say the love they created over time in their arranged marriages is far stronger than the Hollywood driven romantic and lustful fluff so many Americans take for real love. I can't help but believe them, after all their divorce rate is far lower than our own. It's easy to confuse lust for love, and easier still to confuse the magic of the power exchange for love.

Things get even more confusing when defined by the oddities of the D/s dating paradigm. In many ways, we are valued by the amount of experience which we bring to the table. This encourages people to get involved on a casual basis, often with multiple partners. There is often an assumption that intimacy of the D/s kind, whether or not it includes sexual activity, will be a factor very early on in a relationship. Or in the vernacular, that I'm expected to put out pretty darn fast.

Jumping into relationships this quickly can be just as damaging as sleeping around or jumping from one infatuation to another in the vanilla world. Yes, some consider me the prude in our community. I believe the intimacy of the D/s experience is a sacred one, a gift to be given to someone who earns it, not just anyone who asks, or "orders" as the case may be. If you keep changing partners there is always the high, the feeling of new love, new attraction. While that's a great thing, it's not real love, and it's not likely to hold out over the long term. What is lost is the opportunity of the deeper commitment, less exotic, yes, but one where we can be vulnerable on the emotional and spiritual levels, not just the physical ones.

I think it unlikely Dex will ever lean toward me and say "I love you" in the eros sort of way. He may someday love me as his Submissive, with the care and affection obvious in all the couples at House Mermaid. And that, that would be just fine.

Morphing into the Group

This particular evening I have settled in with four couples, most affiliates of House Mermaid and some guests. We bond over Saki's luscious cheese-smothered lasagna and Lady Midnite's purple fruit salad, with sweet drippings glistening when poured over ice cream. Purple and red and pink; juicy and succulent. They are how Lady Midnite sees her Submissive samri, sweet and tasty, and she might just take a big bite.

I wear my silver House Mermaid necklace to dinner, and so I am officially affiliated with the family. I like the feeling of belonging to this witty and energetic group. None of them are bothered by the fact of my writing about them, and perhaps the more exhibitionistic ones relish it. Of course I remind them with a smile that I'm writing about me, not about them, but that's just semantics.

Being with this group at House Mermaid feels different than my experiences with my own community in Vermont. The difference is more than just the few hours away and the established BDSM community there. An important difference is that in my own community I hang around mostly with single people like myself, and while the talk does tease around the politics and the play of BDSM, it's mostly about our lives outside the BDSM experience. With the roomful of couples at House Mermaid, the teasing banter is non-stop, as is the conversation about every sundry aspect of the lifestyle. In some ways, their lives are not outside the BDSM experience, they are one and the same. I have mixed feelings about this. There's a part of me that really doesn't want to talk about this all the time – I don't live it – it's just my sexual orientation.

Yet I can also see how a home space like House Mermaid offers the one place where people can converse with total openness, knowing the house rule of "everything said here stays here" will protect them. (I'm the exception to the rule, but with permission) These couples are more long-term and more lifestyle oriented than most of the people from my Vermont community. The result is a river of wisecracking winding through our various activities from food to play.

It's all pretty wearying to me, but it's not so much the topic of conversation, as that a group, even a group of people I like, can drain me to the point of tears. Dex has been very understanding of this, and sends me to my room periodically to decompress. I relax as much as anyone can in a strange place where someone is bound to wander in eventually. I lay on my bed, writing, an English muffin by my pillow, and the crack of a whip snapping through the hallways. This guest bed is a bondage bed, edged with heavy rings and set so high up that you have to climb a ladder to get on. Dex plans to build stocks into the footboard, forcing the stockee to watch the action, unable to touch. In a cage below, another Submissive will service the one in the stocks, who is as helpless as the one in the cage. On the other hand, my flannel sheets have dogs and cats raining down. They're holding umbrellas and sport an inquisitive expression. It's a strange room.

I love the camaraderie even as I struggle with my own urge to escape to the cave, to a quiet dark place where I'm not "on," where I don't have to charm, to question, to listen, to connect. So far everyone has been very understanding, although who knows what they say about me when I'm not there? If this turns out to be a real family to me, they will accept me as I am, not as the extrovert I appear. Still, I've arranged to visit Dex mostly on weekends where there are no events. I want the time with him more than I want another community. It may mean a few less lasagnas and fruit salads, but I'm hoping that the strand which has connected me to this family will be as strong as the strand of silver around my neck.

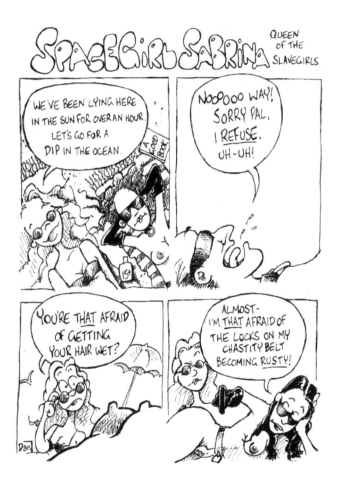

Drunk On Chastity

Some artists take drugs to enhance their artistic or writing expressions. I have chosen to arouse myself, so I will feel the burn of chastity even as I write about it.

All my life I have pursued sex with abandon. Men and women, Dominant and Submissive. In relationship and not. There is a place where I have not yet gone, the place of turning my sexuality over to another person. Yes, I have submitted to Dominants, but they never really owned me. Their interest was more often in making me come as many times as possible, as if it were some kind of testament to their manhood. Deep down though, I wanted them to stop me instead, stop me from coming as many times as possible.

Dex, fortunately, cares little about testaments to his manhood, and has put me on a chastity program. He wants me to learn to control my sexuality, to give up this ultimate pleasure for a greater goal. He made this decision not out of the blue, but because he knew that I needed him to guide me through this dark cave.

Dex sees BDSM as a lifestyle, a paradigm with rules and regs. He once said to me: "BDSM is more than convention, more than protocol, there is a beauty and grace in what we are about, it is much more than simply calling me Sir. Before you can give me your complete self, you must develop enough self-control so to give up total control over your orgasm. It is because we are after a higher calling, a path less traveled."

To me, though, it's mostly about sex. Kinky sex to be sure, but still hovering in the vicinity of the orgasm. There's also a spiritual dimension, of course, but that's not the everyday draw, but rather a summer Sundae's pleasure. We probably won't be doing much in the mystical realm, but Dex is attempting to help me experience D/s independently from sex and orgasm. In exploring it this way, he teaches me awareness of my need for release, not just the orgasmic kind, but the emotional and spiritual kind as well.

I figure I've had plenty of kinky sex in my life and will likely have plenty more in the future, so I can live without it now. Had I wanted to, my vibrator would have provided ten orgasms a day; but I never bothered with that. Now, I want to know what will happen, how I will feel in the absence of the usual, the "pleasure as much as I want" usual. It's not that Dex will never have sex with me or allow me to orgasm, but rather that they are not the main thrust of our spelunking.

He directs me to pleasure myself as much as I wish, but to always stop prior to orgasm. Only he will take me to that place, and it will always be in conjunction with pain. In reading his initial instructions about keeping chaste, I got so turned on that I went directly upstairs and got myself off. Pathetic. Part of the training is in guessing how close I am and being able to stop before I lose control. Yet I did it even knowing I would receive a hard caning as punishment. Maybe once I've actually been caned by Dex, I will take it more seriously, but not now. In a weird way I want the punishment, the reality of it, the memory of it, to keep me on the straight and narrow. I won't believe it until I have that muscle memory.

Since the first failed attempt, I tried three more times, one successful where I was able to stop in time. Dex also had me ice down my pussy between rounds, an act which was profoundly humiliating as well as numbing. The ice burned, and made me feel ever so much more vulnerable.

Even now as I write, I periodically touch myself, trying, hoping I will be able to follow his orders. The very fact they exist makes my cunt quiver. Without orders to be chaste, I might go for weeks or even longer without needing sexual gratification, but having it taken away makes it something I long for, desperately. When I play with my vibrator these days, I do it in short stints. I lay on my stomach because I know it's harder for me to come this way, and maybe that difficulty will prevent me from losing control. My clitoris is engorged by my own pleasure and the pain of stopping. I spread my legs wide and let the air cool me.

There is something which moves me in a very deep level about someone else controlling my orgasm. To have this intimate thing in his hands affects me to my core. I feel my submissive nature acutely, more so than in other submissive pursuits.

I want Dex to tease me, I want him to make me beg, not in mock fun, but for real. I want him to withhold my pleasure so I can truly know what it means to turn it over to him. I want him to make me turn that need over to him, into his hands, literally and figuratively. I want him to torture me, touch me never enough, make me feel the withdrawal as if it is the only thing in the universe. It is in the moment his hand pulls away that I most feel connected to him. I will cry for him; weep, and say anything, hoping that in the end, he is unmoved.

I want to humiliate myself begging him to touch me. I want to be reduced to promising him anything for another moment of his hand on me. I want to suffer pain for any small pleasure allowed. I want to be tied tightly, my legs wide apart so I cannot move, cannot prevent him from manipulating any part of me. I want the core of my being naked.

If there could be more, it would be this. I can think of nothing more humiliating than feeling barbie's hand instead, inside me, touching my most intimate spaces. Dex knows that sexual contact with women is on my "only under duress" list, so this will qualify. What would it be like to have her hand on me, giving me the pleasure I desperately want but in a form so ultimately degrading? How helpless I would feel. How needy. How violated. How naked. There would be my primal self, stripped of everything.

I am ashamed to want these things. I am ashamed even to tell Dex I want them, but if I cannot tell him, who could I tell? If I cannot trust him to take me there, who can I trust? In a way, I look forward to hurting myself, humiliating myself, frustrating myself by another bout with the vibrator which I've come to hate. In a cruel twist, I want to tease myself as much as possible, to keep myself aroused because it makes me acutely aware of his ownership. Dex will truly appreciate this gift, more than anyone could.

I am terrified he will take away my vibrator, and yet I desperately need him to do it. I need him to take it until I am used to the constant feeling of sexual hunger. When I see him next I will give it to him and implore him to take it away, because with it I am too weak.

If only I could wear a real chastity belt, one which would have a cold metal cover over my clitoris. I want to reach down and feel the cold metal, not my own soft wetness. To not be able to reach myself no matter what I do. I am jealous of men because the male chastity belts are simple and utilitarian. The women's belts are wholly impractical, unhygienic, and worthless for anyone who works out. Instead, Dex is getting me a symbolic one, decorative only perhaps, but hopefully it's weight will protect me from myself.

In this gift I give Dex, I am also giving myself a deeper gift, one I have desired for a long time. How will I manage it? Will I fail as often as I have done so far? Or will I find a strength in my commitment to Dex, away and aside from any threats of caning punishments. If I do not have this path to follow, the easy orgasm I could have anytime, where will I travel instead? What strange experiences are in my future because of this turn of the dark corridor? We have only to go forward, and I do, now slowly and each day with a prayer that I am able to take the next step forward.

Stepping Out

I joke sometimes about my lack of modesty, but actually it's quite true. I am vain. Vain about my clothing. Vain about my place in the community. Vain about whoever I partner with, be he Dominant or Submissive. With this in mind, I stepped out to my first Rose & Thorn event with Dex and barbie.

This would be the first time I had ever gone to a Rose & Thorn party (the group I founded) with a Dominant. It may seem bizarre, as it surely did to Dex, but during the last two and a half years, I was primarily exploring my own dominant side. While I submitted with two Dominants, I wasn't in a committed relationship with them. As a leader it seemed perfectly natural to bring my own Submissive along to parties, but far more complicated both on a personal and professional level for a Dominant to bring me.

Having the freedom to be submissive in public was one of the reasons I resigned from leadership, and so I was excited to be finally expressing this side of myself. This was my "coming out," so I was self conscious in a way I had not been before. Before this party, few people even knew who Dex was, not to mention that I was collared to him. Even though Albany is just three hours away, the Vermont community is young in that it has only just started to link up with our neighbors. Interestingly, despite my collar and my sticking with Dex most of the evening, few people realized we were together. Dex had expected everyone to recognize the significance of the collar, but I knew better. Here in Vermont collars are worn just as often for decorative as for commitment reasons. I can imagine that for some people, seeing me as a submissive in public just plain didn't compute.

Dex satisfies my aesthetic sense. He is confident, attractive, and well dressed. Most importantly, he is amiable and open minded, a nice contrast to the many ego-driven Dominants. This quality tells me more about Dex than any amount of posturing would do. He wore the standard black leather outfit, but sparked it up with a leather codpiece (a "pocket" for the penis). I can't begin to guess what codpieces did historically, but they certainly do focus one's attention. Dex's Submissive barbie had brushed her hair into a long golden tress. She wore a shimmering translucent blouse, and white corset which showed off her breasts to perfection. She reflected what many of us imagine of when we think of a traditional Submissive: quiet, gentle, and unassuming.

As we arrived, I reviewed Dex's directions on greeting in my head. In an attempt to keep things simple, he had told me to wait for Dominants to shake hands first, allow my eyes to drop briefly in respect, and then request permission from Dex to speak with them. I was to speak freely to Submissives, as well as switches and people undeclared or undecided, who are all treated as Submissives.

Dex suggested for this first event that I or a Rose & Thorn board member introduce him to everyone at the party, which would help him to identify the orientation of each person. I told him that I certainly didn't know everyone's orientation, and that I doubted that the board did either. This shocked Dex, who considers this prima face information about any scene player.

I explained that I consider one's BDSM orientation to be private, the most intimate expression of a person's elemental self. I would no more ask someone about his or her orientation (unless I was planning on hitting on them) than I would about any other private part of their life. This is not to say that people don't give it up one way or another, but I consider this particular piece of information just one of many. Unfortunately, my paradigm doesn't work for the greeting protocol because you can't treat Dominants differently if you aren't quite sure who they are.

I also have philosophical issues with the idea of treating switches as Submissives. In this world view, people are categorized by the role they would play with Dex, my Dominant. This approach seems backward to me, assuming first a person plays casually, a big assumption. It seems to be a play party orientation parachuted into the social setting, focusing on orientation rather than on who anyone is as a person. I also feel uncomfortable making the choice of someone's orientation for them, even if only for politeness purposes. I know a lot of switches, including myself, who would find this offensive.

Dex also told me that if I don't know someone's orientation, I shouldn't be doing the huggy kissy with them. This also suggests to me a hierarchy in that people who don't declare themselves one thing or another are less worthy of affection. This paradigm just doesn't work for me. I hug people I care about, and don't hug people I don't care about. To me, their D/s identity is irrelevant.

I found my attempts to follow greeting protocol mostly unsuccessful as I tried desperately to remember each person's orientation even as they ran up and hugged me. I got confused when we were talking to people in a small group when I couldn't be sure if technically they were speaking to me or not, not to mention what I was supposed to do when I was greeted from across the room. Dex did not punish me for these things, presumably because it was my first attempt, or maybe he simply realized the difficulty of making this protocol work in this situation.

I never did ask Dex for permission to speak to anyone because none of the three known Dominants greeted me formally, and when they did speak to me it was in a casual sense later on in the party which was well past the greeting stage. Sometimes it was a group situation where they weren't actually speaking "to me." By this time I was no longer tethered to Dex by the six-foot rule, and I had no idea where he was or how I would manage excusing myself to ask permission to converse, when we were only exchanging a few words in the first place. In a group where traditional protocol is observed (and where a big hugfest wasn't going on) it might be easier to follow these rules.

As we moved into the demonstration I have to admit a fair bit of pride about the caliber of play which Dex represented, such as it reflected on me as well. God knows I've seen a jillion demonstrations, and I had prepared to assume an interested expression while my mind wandered in far-away fields. Dex's demonstration was superior both on the practical as well as the emotional levels. It wasn't just his skill with the single tail, but his obvious connection with barbie. I was particularly impressed that unlike many who espouse one technique as the "right" way, he described several ways to do things, and explained that the important thing is not following one technique or another, but safe play.

After a short informational discussion, he warmed barbie up with a moose flogger and a tomcat, preparing her skin for the more intense single tail. He spent a couple of songs single-tailing her shoulders and tush in alternating figure eights, and finished with an aphrodisiac teasing of the nipples, which acted as an erotic cooldown. Barbie looked beautiful even as she fell into subspace with barely a murmur. How courageous to have bared herself in a crowd of strangers, not just her body but her submission. The most poignant moment was at the end when he took her down from the St. Andrew's Cross, and held her close for long moments. The room was dead silent, and instead of the usual raucous applause, watchers tip-toed out, leaving the room hushed, the two of us huddled around barbie who sat dazed with post subspace languor.

As I explored Dex's world, I sometimes did things which weren't necessarily in alignment with my own world view. In general I feel this is a good thing, as long as it isn't in conflict with my spiritual path. Another way to put this is that Dex collared my body and my submissive spirit, but my soul will always belong to me and God.

If I've moved from the most superficial, my vanity, to the most profound, my relationship with God, it is because at a deeper levels they are one and the same. My vanity is an expression of the pride I have in my self. Yes, I am full of myself, full of the many gifts strewn along my path. Each one I lift up, and walk on to the next in joyful, and occasionally vain expectation.

So, What Do You Feel About all This?

Years ago when I was tumbling around in my turbulent twenties, my counselor would listen to me ramble a bit, then she'd say "but what do you *feel* about this?" I was distracted. I was dissembling. I didn't know what I felt and even if I did, I couldn't put it into words.

When I read over my experience with House Mermaid so far, I heard a little voice asking me what was I feeling about all this. The thing about new experiences is that there's a lot to write about, even if you aren't really feeling much at all. It's still easy to distract and dissemble in the course of writing an entertaining story. I write about my relationship with Dex or barbie. My public personae; His; Ours. Attempts to emulate, sometime failures at communication. Trying on new philosophies like trying on bathing suits. This and that.

Yet the voice got it right. Did I feel anything about all this? Or was it just something I couldn't yet articulate?

First the facts. I'm finding the whole experience intriguing. It's fun to peek into another life and try it on for a little while, knowing I can take it off anytime. Although I am trying to live it, not just play at it. It's the method acting thing Marlon Brando made popular, where you don't just act, but live the character. Knowing that it's part of the gestalt, it's easier to do things I don't necessarily want to do. Yet the thing I've enjoyed the most has not been the actual experience of affiliating with House Mermaid, but the writing about it. Considering that my submissive muse is as powerful as my writer's muse, it's no surprise.

The connection has been superficial so far, presumably because most of our activities emphasize the "form" of BDSM. To Dex, BDSM is an art form. He is an architect, focusing on the grace of the experience. He is exquisitely attuned to the subtleties, from greeting a fellow Dominant to the twist of his wrist on the elkskin flogger. It is not unlike watching someone paint a portrait. He pulls together a particular brand of oil paint, the perfect violet color, the detailing paintbrush, canvas hand-stretched on the frame, the spot lighting. When all this comes together, there is House Mermaid, Dex's artistic expression.

I am learning a lot about art, but are we making a connection? Are my emotions engaged? Is my spirit flying? Probably not.

While I appreciate the beauty in form, I care little for symbolism or ceremony, and much of the subtlety is lost on me. It's sad really, because I know he'd really like me to "get" it. I hail from a spiritual orientation, searching for meaning and connection in a community often cluttered with protocol, fashion, and an affection for toys. Sometimes so much affection that the actual experience, the union, becomes secondary.

I want to feel the magic of spirituality, the mystery of sexual attraction, the seductive eroticism of slipping into subspace. I want a moment in the darkest dark when I whisper "I love you," and then wonder if I really spoke those words, or just imagined them, pixies dancing off in a wink of shimmering wings and tiny flying feet.

We're not quite there yet, and maybe that will never be the essence of our connection. Just this morning Dex and I had a discussion about tightlacing corsets, a conversation illustrating the elemental difference in our approaches. As I knew he would, he took the traditional view, which endorses tightlacing because there is no medical damage to the body. He sees corsets as a construct of the lifestyle, a visible construction which by its very nature reflects certain beliefs and practices. That is certainly true, but then those certain beliefs and practices aren't much in alignment with mine so it's no big surprise that tightlacing doesn't work for me either.

I believe the body is a temple, the physical expression of my spiritual nature. It is something sacred, something to be cherished. Tightlacing forces the body to become a stylized form, changing the organization of the internal organs. It prevents you from breathing deeply, prohibits exercise as well as other activities. Breathing is more than just about staying alive, it connects us to our bodies as well as to our inner spiritual selves. While moving one's organs around may not be medically dangerous (as long as it's done correctly which it often isn't), tightlacing interferes with the integrity of the body on the most fundamental level. Some might feel that Dex is the Dominant and if he tells me to wear a tightlacing corset, I should wear it. But this isn't a my way/your way disagreement, it is far more fundamental to who I am as a person. Fundamental in a way which isn't up for discussion.

Aside from our generally disagreeing about this particular issue, I think it also bothered Dex that I wrote about these beliefs, because they were in conflict with the party line. Fortunately for me, being in conflict with the party line has never bothered me any. Fortunately for us, we agreed to disagree.

Are these paradigms incompatible long-term? Probably. Still, I can enjoy Dex's style for the art it is. I enjoy the philosophical banter, although it is sometimes tiring to have to defend myself to someone who finds so many of my ideas incomprehensible. I suppose he sometimes feels the same way about defending his ideas; God knows I tell him exactly what I think about just about everything.

The challenge is not in whether or not our beliefs are in alignment, but how to answer the question "what do you feel about all this?"

The truth is, I don't feel much of anything. It's not the same as being 20 years old and in shock from being tossed about like a bit of flotsam. There are many things I feel passionately about, but form isn't one of them. I'm not sure I would even want an emotional connection with Dex because it would certainly make things far less compartmentalized, far less neat. I'm not sure my heart is ready in any case. It has been two years since I loved someone, and it is only now that I feel I might love again. I can feel my heart opening up like a fluffy chick pecking out of her shell. Tender, very tender, but persistent.

Dex does not offer the "erotica mystica" I have written about, and yet, neither is he a weekend warrior offering only casual play. It is his unique and visionary approach which draws me to him. I may not feel anything at the moment, and I may not even mind it. Down the road a bit maybe there will be a frisson, and we will move to the next level, or maybe not. Either way, we will both have experienced exactly what we wanted to, and that's the only thing which matters.

It Ain't Entirely a Bowl of Cherries

It's been a few months getting to know Dex, made up of a few weekends, various social occasions, phone calls and plenty of e-mail. I have learned a lot about his lifestyle, and he's learned a lot about mine.

One of the challenges has been that Dex and I have not found a lot of common ground in our approach. From what I have observed, Dex seems primarily interested in BDSM as a construct, while I focus on the emotional and spiritual connection. Dex doesn't agree with me on this, describing his experience in this way: "My soul is extended to barbie as she leaves her body and flies. Where she goes I do not know, only the greatest feeling in the world is when I take her off the cross and she crumbles safely into my arms." I was surprised to hear him say something like this since our interaction so far hasn't even hinted at anything like this. It made me more than a little sad to hear what I'd missed out on.

On the other hand, I wonder if it's not so much my missing out on anything, but rather that while we may be using the same words, we mean entirely different things. Our discussions about both philosophical and personal issues have been an ongoing challenge because we speak such different languages.

An interesting example of this apparent difference in styles manifested a few weeks ago when I was doing some processing with Moby, my ex-partner. I figured Dex might be concerned because Moby had been the love of my life, so if anyone would be a threat, Moby would be. I told Dex that Moby and I were not considering getting back together, only seeking some closure on loose emotional ends. The emotional stuff wasn't Dex's concern, however. His question was about whether Moby was a Dominant, which would make him a threat because while more than one Dominant can reside in a BDSM house, ultimately only one Dominant can preside. Dex's second concern was the fact that Moby had not followed protocol in approaching me. It turns out neither of these issues were germane because Moby had been submissive to me, but I couldn't help but wonder why Dex was so focused on the protocol of my experience when I was just trying to get through it.

Our challenges have not only been theoretical, however. One of the practical issues is that Dex and I have had so little time in private. I suspect his relationship with me has to take a back seat because he has so many balls in the air: work, hobbies and House Mermaid, not to mention his relationship with barbie.

Yet, it's more than just logistics. Dex and barbie have an agreement that his private time with me whether play or not, is restricted to House Mermaid. With the lively social schedule there, little time remains for personal interaction. Since the agreement doesn't allow him to spend time with me alone when he's here in Vermont, and because he doesn't practice BDSM via phone or e-mail, our options are limited to my visits to the house. As of the moment, we have only spent one hour alone which was during our introductory session. I kept hoping things would change and I'd get more time to connect with Dex, but so far it hasn't happened.

This kind of agreement is different than my previous poly relationships where the person with the long-term partner generally did not play in their own home, whether it was me or them. We felt our homes were sacred ground for our primary love relationships, and that overt boundaries both on emotional and pragmatic levels were a good thing. In general, we were also experienced in the process of negotiating private time, leaving only the practical details to work out. I think had I known the House Mermaid limitations would be so binding (so to speak), Dex and I might have negotiated a different kind of relationship. This was a good lesson for me in knowing what questions to ask.

Another area wherein I failed to ask the right questions was how barbie wanted to relate to me. I think I assumed it would be like my previous polysomething relationships where I was on friendly, if not intimate terms with my lover's partner or spouse. Admittedly, I think I may have expected more than "friendly, if not intimate terms" from barbie because of our unique situation. Unfortunately barbie's life is also full up with work, hobbies and House Mermaid, not to mention her relationship with Dex. I soon realized that a relationship with me was not on her priority list, which surprised me. I had assumed she'd be very interested in me, both as a sister Submissive and someone who was writing about her life.

I decided not to pressure her because she has a lot on her emotional plate without me adding to it. Since barbie and I are so different, I didn't really expect us to become buddy Submissives, but it has been a bit disappointing. She and Dex have been together for three years in a committed relationship, and although they sometimes top or bottom with other people, with Dex always controlling the scene, they haven't engaged in committed long-term relationships with anyone else. In some ways I am a "transition" Submissive, a catalyst for them to learn about being in a poly relationship. Dex is her first Master, as well as a Master who has been entirely committed to her for three years. Since he has decided to bring in two more Submissives to House Mermaid, barbie's world is definitely changing. It's sure understandable she would have mixed feelings about all of it. I wonder how much of all this affected her relationship with me.

 When I look over all the things I've experienced with House Mermaid, it's a wildly mixed bag of different stories. Although I have very much enjoyed the experience of being affiliated to House Mermaid, there are some parts that don't seem to be a good fit. I wonder if those parts might be the ones which make it difficult to take the next step into the year-long training collar. I'm still thinking on it all, and keeping an open mind until we get to the negotiation. Either way, Dex and I both have a lot to learn.

Closure

One of the interesting patterns in my life is that the ideals to which I've made formal commitments often didn't amount to much, while many things I chose on an organic basis became lifelong commitments. For example, the last time I made a formal commitment to my Submissive, our relationship ended a year later. His choice? My choice? It doesn't matter, only that it happened. Then again fifteen years ago I started working out. I liked how the feeling of physical strength transformed to spiritual groundedness. I hadn't made any commitments to anyone, much less my aerobics teacher, but fifteen years later this is one of the foundations of my life. It was an organic commitment, chosen day-by-day until it became an inextricable part of my life.

So when I started thinking about making a commitment to a training collar, I felt pretty indecisive. Such a commitment is daunting. A year long. On the good side, Dex is dependable, kind, and very knowledgeable. The family at House Mermaid is tight knit and supportive. They say the best predictor of future behavior is past behavior, so I have a pretty good idea of what I could have expected.

What has been a challenge is the distance and logistics. Two and a half hours away may not seem far, but far enough to mean no dropping by for a cuppa or a quick spanky. Far enough that with little other interaction besides those one or two weekends a month, I might be tempted to wander into other territories.

On the heart side, there is my lack of connection, of resonance with what I have experienced. I don't know why this is, but it's probably that a formal BDSM lifestyle is simply not a good fit for me. I didn't really expect to feel moved at the deepest level because I knew Dex's style was very different than mine. I had hoped to feel more than I did. Surely, to make such a commitment there should be something more than interested speculation?

I am a passionate person. Passionate about my "platform" as Dex puts it. Passionate about experiencing D/s with every bit of my body, mind, and soul. But I haven't the passion for this; this Master, this house, this experience. I worry that someone at House Mermaid might take this personally, but it is no criticism. In fact, I have only respect and admiration for everything I have seen there.

There were many experiences at House Mermaid I found memorable. The thing that touched me the deepest was the feeling of ownership. It was fleeting, noticed at obscure times between odd moments. A shadow passing over me like a passing ghost, hard to grasp and forge into sentences. Perhaps it will grow longer, just as the day stretches into evening, and I will discover the true meaning of commitment to one Master.

While it was sometimes challenging to have to defend my beliefs as well as to understand Dex's philosophy, I was energized by our debates about different aspects of the lifestyle. Rarely do I have the opportunity to observe and deliberate without anyone taking it personally. This experience has changed my own practice in subtle ways. There were parts of the protocol which brought a certain sense of stability and security. I loved the feeling of being cared for and part of a committed relationship. There is a safety there which gave me space to explore in other ways, and I'll miss that.

It's hard to separate Dex from his BDSM style, and I wonder how different this experience might have been with a different Dominant. I probably will not know until I have something for comparison, and which might be years from now. For the moment, I feel satisfied with what I learned, and blessed to have been taken into their lives in such good faith.

The writing experience has been different for me as well. While I have often written about people in my life, those actual people were often obscured in the story. With this series on House Mermaid, the house members read my writing as it emerged, and Dex was fully engaged with my writing, and in fact had limited editorial control. I wonder if there is a fundamental conflict of interest between the writer as writer and the writer as Submissive. There is an awareness of balancing my writing muse and my Submissive muse, both of which are equally strong. My question is not in which is more important, but whether one can ever be totally conscious of an experience when it is immediately poured into a "story truth." Something like the difference between being in subspace, and writing about it. One is experiential, one is analytical. Words can only approximate the experience.

I've read that in certain scientific examinations, particles appear to be waves or particles depending on what equipment you use to examine them, something which would seem to be mutually exclusive. Could my observation of the experience, and of my writing have affected what was occurring? There is no way to know, and in this case one could not have existed without the other.

Regardless of the "reality" of the experience, for the first time in two years, I feel ready to love again. It may be coincidence, but then not believing in coincidence, I wonder what my experience at House Mermaid contributed to this loosening of the steel band which was so tightly bound to my heart. I can feel my next partner moving toward me on the spiritual plane. Instead of imaging a list of traits, this time I sense someone who is a vibrational match for me. Someone with whom I can explore both the world and the BDSM world, hand in hand. Perhaps it will become clear as I move into my next relationship, perhaps this time through an organic commitment begun with small things, and growing to take both of us into each other's lives, inextricably.

Part IV
Relationships & Community

Just a few years back I was pretty much just me, just Sadie. Then came Rose & Thorn, writing, and a whole different perspective which you can read about in my first piece of this section: *Think Globally, Spank Locally*. My life may look pretty much the same on the outside, but my attitude has broadened radically. Read on to see how.

Think Globally, Spank Locally - also known as Our Community is more than one big Spank-a-Thon

In the nearly three years I spent with Ryan, he taught me a great deal about BDSM play. From his lighthearted sense of humor to his gigantic toy bag, each visit was a dessert of delights. Sadly, his move to Florida in 1999 left me adrift, and so prompted me to start Rose & Thorn, an act which would change my life. When he returned after four years, I thought we might pick up where we had left off. To my surprise, I discovered that while Ryan was just as intelligent and sexy, I had surpassed him, literally and figuratively.

It wasn't just Ryan that I had outgrown. Before Rose & Thorn, I was just another kinky girl. Now I see what was invisible to me before: the groups, the leaders, the events, the publications, the writers, and the activists. We work at many purposes, from education to spiritual enlightenment, from legal activism to just plain fun; but the community is far more than just a bunch of people spanking their hands out each weekend. We form a cohesive organism with a life of its own, one that may have been active in the big cities for years, but which is revolutionary to much of the rest of the country, especially rural areas like Vermont where I make my home.

I've come to believe that community is the key to credibility and validation by the larger world. Seeing so many players like myself - with jobs and kids and homes - helped me recognize that BDSM is not a dark secret of people on the edge of society. Rather, it is a valid and creative way of expressing our sexuality. This knowledge is critical in our self acceptance, and helps create circumstances where vanilla people can learn about us as well. More importantly, our institutions create a place where we can grow, learn, and connect in a safe space. It is these institutions, as well as activists and writers that shine the light of reason and acceptance on us.

It was in this context that I found myself reading an open letter from writers and activists Cleo Dubois and Fakir Musafar, asking for support and prayers for author Patrick Califia who's been having a rough time. Early on when far less people were aware of my writing, I asked Patrick to do an interview with me, and he kindly responded with over 8,000 words, the longest interview I've received. This was even more amazing knowing that his fibromyalgia made typing painful, and that he was not paid one red cent for those 8,000 words. One might even say that this very selfless devotion to the community has in part put him in his present financial crunch.

Because of my feelings toward his generosity, I forwarded the letter to a few of my favorite discussion groups. I received two kinds of responses to the request. One was "Who the heck is Patrick Califia?" and the other was "How can you be asking for support for an individual when we are possibly facing a war with Iraq?"

These comments surprised me, but my response to both was the same: Patrick is a well known BDSM writer, but he is far more than just another kinky player draped in black leather.

Gary Switch, contributing editor to Prometheus magazine says that, "Califia is simply the most intelligent, most radical, most provocative, most passionate, best-writing advocate for sexual liberation that we have." Cleo Dubois adds that "Patrick has been an outspoken opponent of censorship of BDSM literature. Through essays and other writings like those collected in Public Sex, he has challenged prejudice against our community and expanded our sense of who we are to include spirituality and activism as well as sexuality."

What I find particularly interesting about Patrick is that he represents a commonality with my vanilla lesbian friends. They tell me that prior to his transformation to a man, Pat Califia (as he was known then) was busy shaking things up in the lesbian camp as well. I sure can see why. Every fringe group seeks credibility from the larger community, and people like Pat Califia muddy the waters of a lesbian platform aiming to mainstream lesbian identity.

They also told me the story of how the Gay/Lesbian/Bisexual/Transgendered (GLBT) world went a bit awry when Pat became Patrick a few years ago. By transforming to a man, Patrick in some ways repudiated those who had nurtured him. My friend Dana reflects this approach when she tells me that, "being a lesbian is more than sleeping with a woman, it's a whole political identity." Another friend Mia adds that, "I can't tell you how many times I have heard that I am not a real lesbian because I fucked men over 15 years ago, or because I have male friends." In some ways I understand this approach because the BDSM community is in the same boat, in fact far further from the shore of acceptance. I have had similar feelings about some BDSM authors I know who are no longer active in the lifestyle. It felt a little bit like they had invalidated the meaning of their words if they didn't believe them enough to continue being part of the lifestyle. So in a way I can understand those same feelings in the lesbian community, and can just imagine the reaction of the gay and transgendered communities that he moved into.

My response then to those questions posed to me is this: Patrick is a visionary of our community, regardless of his orientation or gender. I might even say that because he does not fit into a nice neat mold of male, female, lesbian, gay, bi, Dominant, Submissive, Switch or whatever, he can speak a truth that only someone of ambiguous orientation can. Patrick is not the only visionary that we have, but he is an important one, one who has fought for us in a thousand ways that most of us will never have to. Straight leatherfolk may not be as aware of his work because of its focus on GLBT, but his words, whether oriented toward that audience or not, only emphasize the importance of pansexual unity.

Secondly, I do not believe that we should allow the spectre of warfare to distract us from our continuing struggle for acceptance. We are beholden to support our community's leaders, emotionally and spiritually, and sometimes even financially. We must do this because it is not the private players who are making the world a safer place to express our orientation; it's people like Patrick who are doing that work. This work is as important as war, because when the fighting is over, we will still be living in a culture that represses sexuality, and practically criminalizes radical sexuality. There will always be some political or economic or personal situation to distract us. In fact, I might venture to say that the worse the economic situation is, the more important it is for us to support the writers, leaders, and activists who have devoted their lives to our cause, when they could have chosen a much safer, much better-paying career.

In watching this drama unfold, I see my own experience reflected in the larger community. You may choose to play strictly on your own time, and that's fine. But I ask you to consider a different paradigm. Just as we are asked to think globally and act locally to make our world a better place, I ask you to consider thinking globally and spanking locally. Our community, our lifestyle, is more than just play that goes on behind closed doors. We are entering mainstream culture, and through this freedom many who were afraid to explore BDSM can now do so freely. Because of organizations like the National Coalition for Sexual Freedom (NCSF), I know that if I were to ever face a backlash because of my writing, someone would be there to stand up with me.

The story here is that it's not about Patrick, it's about what he represents to each of us, whether we are aware of it or not. It's about the National Coalition for Sexual Freedom and the Leather Leadership Conference. It's about writers like John Warren and Laura Antoniou, who write for us and for the masses. It's about the BDSM group in your town, and the volunteer leaders who provide a safe environment for all of us. It's about giant events like the Folsom Street Fair and the New York S/M Film Festival, and about small events like the munch last Friday night. All of these are tentacles that are slowly bringing BDSM into a place of credibility and acceptance.

Are you wondering what I want from you? There is something, but it's not what you might think. I'm not asking you to march in a leather pride parade or go lobby for BDSM acceptance in Washington. What I am asking you to do is make your daily actions count; that is - spank locally. Come out to the people who know you and dispel the aura of secrecy around what we do. Keeping secrets perpetuates fear. Educate yourself and share your knowledge, especially with novices. Get involved with your local BDSM group and offer to help out. Support our authors by buying their books. Join one of the leather groups who fight for our rights. If the media portrays a BDSM players as dangerous whackos, write a letter of complaint. If a writer, a leader, or just another scene person touches your life - tell them. Fighting the good fight can be a thankless job and a little thank you can make all the difference.

Now that my eyes have been opened to this interdependent web, I cannot be that Submissive who thought Ryan was the be all and end all of Dominants. Nor can I be that person who thinks only of her own pleasure, either on a personal or a political level. Today I am proud to be part of our kinky society and that is why I write, because these words reach far further than I ever could in person, from my home in Vermont to London, and even to Israel. They have become part of the mosaic of our community, one strand of a powerfully strong and flexible network. This strength will be critical as we move into the next phase of our community's development which I hope and dream will allow all of us to explore freely without fear.

I still had a great time playing with Ryan, but when that was over, I took his hand and showed him what's happening outside our bedroom window, quietly now, but like a wind rising into a mighty storm.

BDSM Relationships: Vanilla with a Dash of Kink, or a Whole Different Animal?

Once upon a time when I dated vanilla men, I went for the tough looking types. I may not have known what BDSM was, but I knew what I wanted and this was the only way I could get it. What I got was a lot of rough sex with a few spankings, a few blindfolds, and a few ties to the bed. It wasn't until I entered the wide wide world of BDSM that I discovered how different an animal it is.

Many players think of BDSM as spice for their love life, or just a different style of lovemaking, like bisexual play versus heterosexual play. But even these are still variations on the vanilla model of relationships. I have observed several fundamental differences in the way that BDSM relationships play out. I believe that it is a completely different paradigm, just as the experience of having relationships in cyberspace is a radical departure from thousands of years of having relationships in person. There are also many things in common: love, respect, trust, commitment, connection; the things that most people yearn for. So, what's so different? This article will look at some of those differences and outline a model for a unique type of relationship.

The main challenge in defining the BDSM relationship is that you can argue down just about any definition because it's so difficult to measure relationships quantitatively. You might talk about the "power exchange," but then of course that very same dynamic is present in many vanilla relationships. You might bring up bondage, or sadism; but even those are present in traditional relationship at one level or another. My approach to BDSM has to do with the quality and intensity of the commitment to these things, a qualitative approach, and one that puts BDSM on a continuum with vanilla relationships; related in the sense that all relationships are about connection, but clearly different. While each person's definition will be unique to their approach to relationships, most will agree that relationships where the participants define the dynamic as BDSM are practicing the elements of Bondage, Discipline, Dominance, Submission, Sadism, and Masochism at a far more intense level.

So here is my own paradox - that Vanilla and BDSM exist on the same continuum, but in many ways are qualitatively different. Despite these challenges, I might argue that while a handy definition may elude me, I know it when I see it.

Open Communication is Not an Option

Many vanilla couples go for years before ever sharing fantasies with each other. In contrast, BDSM couples often exchange checklists of their most intimate sexual interests and health issues before ever engaging in play. I even signed health disclosure and consent forms with one Dominant. This level of communication changes the way people relate and interact before they have intimate relations. It can also cause problems for people who cannot talk openly about their sexuality. This kind of discussion about sexuality is equally important in the vanilla world, but not only can be easily disregarded, but in fact is often frowned upon. Disregarding communication in the BDSM sphere can lead to more than just hurt feelings, it can lead to physical harm.

More Variety and Exploration of Non-Traditional Types of Eroticism

My sister has told me of her eight hour lovemaking sessions with her paramour, but it's all basically in the domain of vanilla sex. She's a bit of a bawdy girl like myself, so she may include lingerie, anal sex, oral sex, and other "traditional" sexual flavors. But no where in all that lingerie, anal sex, and oral sex is there a power exchange. No where is there the kind of implements you'll find hanging in my closet: floggers, fleece-lined cuffs, pinwheels, and more. It's not just about the equipment, but our approach to using that equipment.

BDSM relationships by definition include a wider variety of relationship styles and orientations. Bisexuality, homosexuality, heterosexuality, polygamy, polyamory, and open relationships are common and discussed freely. Then there is the Bondage, Discipline, Dominance, Submission, Sadism, and Masochism of the BDSM panorama. Unlike the vanilla world we are commonly in contact with cross-dressers, transgendered persons, and people with specialized fetishes.

Unlike my sister who has been making love essentially the same way for 20 years, we have expectations of continually exploring new territories.

More Focus on Non-Sexual Modes of Intimate Relations

Much of BDSM is about sex, but much of it is not. Lots of exploration occurs in alternative ways of experiencing our body, mind, and spirit, from body modification to masochistic surrender to the "flow" of Dom and Subspace. Orgasms are nice, but we can have those anytime. BDSM offers a unique means to connect with another human being.

Freedom to Express Our Orientation without Fear

While all these variations on the BDSM theme do occur in the vanilla world, they are often explored secretly, with a sense of shame, and with an awareness that these activities are considered abuse or mental illness. Only within our own relationships and community can we speak freely and express our BDSM orientation in our own way, without fear.

More Structure

BDSM relationships have an inherent structure that may or not be present in vanilla relationships. The Dominant/Submissive form is a yin/yang of giving and receiving power. The power exchange may occur with vanilla couples, but it is an unstated and covert operation. In contrast, we revel in making this exchange overt, often through written contracts. Whether it be a 24/7 Master/slave relationship or just an hour of topping someone after breakfast, the roles are clearly delineated.

A Greater Vulnerability

There is a great vulnerability in loving someone, but turning over your body and mind to another human being requires a greater vulnerability, a unique faith. When we give up control over our selves, we experience something that has no parallel in the vanilla paradigm. (except maybe in the army.) This also means that when our relationships fail, the fallout can be more devastating. It's one thing to make love with someone you hardly know, where the biggest risk is a sexually transmitted disease or a pregnancy. BDSM relationships not only absorb those risks, but add the emotional risks of being totally helpless, or totally in control.

Burning Hot and Sizzling Cold
　　We all know vanilla friends who fall in love, do crazy things, then discover a few months down the road that they made a radical mistake. Love does indeed make us see people the way we want to see them. The dynamics of BDSM add another layer to this complex dynamic. It's common for BDSM relationships to burn as hot as the love infatuation, then sputter out even colder. Part of this has to do with the fact that novices who have fantasized about a BDSM experience their whole life often go a little crazy their first time out of the gate. But even experienced players can lose sight of their rational mind when trying out new types of BDSM play. The experience of exploring a new part of your Dominant or Submissive nature is a form of infatuation in itself, sometimes causing us to bite off way more than we can chew, or mistake those wildly new sensations as love or commitment. Maintaining a relationship is hard enough, but maintaining it in the BDSM context is a heck of a bear.

Exhibitionism & Learning By Example
　　There is a much higher level of exhibitionism in the BDSM culture than in the vanilla one. Only a few minority cultures such as the gay and swingers parties in the vanilla culture even allow for, much less encourage this kind of behavior. The vanilla model is one of keeping sex in the bedroom, in private. In contrast, we can attend play parties designed to allow us to interact in front of an audience. We also have the opportunity to learn from mentors at play parties and in private, in a way that rarely occurs in the vanilla sphere.

More Poseurs

　　I've often wondered why so many players in the scene who do not seem to be well grounded emotionally. For someone with shaky self esteem or self image, BDSM is a powerful construct on which to base a new personality. You will find Dominants who started out as pretty nice people (although maybe a bit insecure), dress in yards of black leather in order to gain a respect that they did not previously engender. On the Submissive side, being taken care of by someone can provide a sense of self esteem and identity that may not be available to them as a regular Joe or Jane. While there are certainly lots of people in the vanilla world who use their work or hobbies to construct an identity, there's not much risk with some fool pretending they're a CEO when they're not. There is a risk with both Dominants and Submissives who do not know themselves well enough to play safely or engage in relationships.

Greater Risk and Greater Payoff
With physical and emotional vulnerability comes higher risk. We risk our bodies being damaged, being outed, and having our heart broken in strange ways that we are not equipped to handle. Of course even vanilla people have their hearts broken, but our social structure and culture supports and even glamorizes the broken heart. There is no rulebook in the public arena (notwithstanding books on BDSM) that helps a slave manage the unique pain of being dumped by a Master who he worshipped. Not only are we mostly on our own when it comes to recovering from failed BDSM relationships, but we often cannot share the unique issues of our relationships with our vanilla friends, who simply cannot understand what it is that we do.

On the good side, the rewards can be extraordinary. Not just to love, but to fly. Not just to have intimacy, but to see right into another's soul. To trust as you have never trusted before; to be trusted as you have never been trusted before. Our relationships may be more work and more risk, but the payoff is an incomparable experience.

How to Spot a Dominant at Ten Paces

I spotted Ronin at the munch. Tall with long black hair in a ponytail. Dark eyes with a faintly Asian cast. Buttery leather jacket with silver snakeskin boots. Despite myself, my hand trembled as I took my Kahlua from the bartender. Yes, Ronin looks exactly like the Dominant of my dreams. Confident, assertive, mysterious.

Ronin looks like the Dominant of my dreams, but may well not be. It's easy to be fooled by beautiful hair, fabulous leathers, or a confident attitude. The bottom line is that there is no way to spot a Dominant at ten paces! Unfortunately many Submissives, and particularly novices, are impressed by these superficial things, making it easy for Dominant fakers. Anyone can learn to swing a flogger, talk in BDSMspeak, and wear 13 pounds of leather; but these do not a Dominant make.

If you want a quality partner you'll have to take some time and get to know them. In some ways, choosing a good Dominant is similar choosing a good partner in general. In others it's quite different because of the unique style of our relationships. They key difference is that when we go into subspace, we make ourselves vulnerable in ways that we may never do with a vanilla partner.

This makes the D/s relationship far riskier and we must take extra care when choosing partners. Here are some things to look for, to avoid, and to ignore in your search for a quality Dominant.

A Dominant Is...

Respect

A quality Dominant shows respect to Submissives, and to everyone. He or she asks questions about your life, listens to the answers, and doesn't put you down. One man I spoke to recently referred to my writing (which I consider my best gift) as "your little columns." If you hadn't guessed already, I didn't go out with him.

Balance

A quality Dominant keeps a balance between their vanilla and BDSM lives. They can talk about their family, pets, other things that have nothing to do with BDSM. They have a sense of humor about the lifestyle, and don't take themselves too seriously. Avoid Dominants with a chip on their shoulder, or who cannot hold a job or keep friends. Especially avoid people who complain about their ex partners or about everyone else in the scene. One day you will be the ex and they will be bitching about you.

Communication

A quality Dominant needs to be able to access their emotions, and articulate them. If they are the stereotypical guy who can't express their emotional side, they will not be able to support your emotional side when the time comes. If they can't control their temper, or they make a big drama out of life, they will be too self-directed to take care of you. One Dominant I know changes the subject when I talk about sad or angry emotions. I don't mind so much when it's about small things, but this tells me that I couldn't depend on him if I were really upset about something.

Consistency

A quality Dominant is as good as their word. If they say they'll show up at 6 PM, they show up. If you are going to trust this person with your body and possibly your heart, you need to know that they will come through. A sometime Dominant is not an effective Dominant.

Depth

A quality Dominant recognizes that D/s relationships have several dynamics that are very different, and sometimes far more complex than vanilla ones. Because of this, he or she should have a better understanding of human nature than the average Joe or Jane. Messing with subspace is a heavy experience. My friend Kim has commented that, "to live a present life you have to understand human nature. But to be a successful Dominant, you have to really get it at a much deeper level." Doing it with a shallow or superficial person makes for a shallow and superficial experience.

Competency

A quality Dominant does not need to know how to use every toy in the toy box, but they do need to be motivated to learn. A novice should not be doing high-end play like whipping, fire play, or knife play without a mentor to guide them. They should be knowledgeable about how to avoid sexually transmitted diseases, and have an awareness of first aid. They know that reading and fantasizing about BDSM is not the same thing as doing it. My friend Sarah adds that "a good Dom acknowledges that he's not the be-all end-all of information. He encourages you to find information about BDSM from many sources."

Pacing

A quality Dominant doesn't hit on you during the first date, and doesn't discourage you from dating other people until you are ready to make a commitment. They know that a good relationship takes time and that there's no need to rush in or glom onto you. They also don't try to "make" you submit before you have given permission to go ahead.

References

A quality Dominant is known by someone. A novice may not have BDSM references, but everyone has friends and family. If they are totally in the closet and can't even offer a vanilla reference then they might not be a good person to get involved with. Being "known" in the scene doesn't guarantee that a person is a good Dominant, but they will probably be a safe Dominant. I know plenty of Dominants who have great reputations because of their technical knowledge, but have little to offer when it comes to the complexities of a real relationship.

A Quality Dominant Isn't...

Lord This and Mistress That

In the days of the Old Guard, a Dominant had to "earn" their leather vest. Anyone who wore it could be considered a safe and experienced player. Today, anyone can call themselves Lady Bigcheese or Master Bigshot. Author Jay Wiseman writes in his article "Ten Tips for the Novice, Single, Heterosexual, Submissive Woman" of a submissive friend who "has concluded that there is also a strong inverse relationship between how many titles a man awards himself and how good a dominant he is." Similarly if they make an "entrance" a la Scarlet O'Hara or claim relationships with many well-known scene personalities, they lose points on the respect-o-meter. Ignore the titles and look at the person.

Cheating on their Partner
   A Dominant who will cheat on their partner, be it spouse or other relationship, will also cheat on you. I believe in Safe Sane and Consensual (SSC), and cheating on your partner is not consensual. A Dominant who lies is not a safe Dominant.

Toy Obsessions
   Dominants who obsess about their toy collections send the message that BDSM is about the toys. It's not. A quality Dominant does not need equipment to dominate, only a powerful and creative mind. Not to mention those who dangle multiple toys off their belt, especially when they aren't playing.

Horndog on the Prowl
   Many novice Dominants or vanilla horndogs view Submissives as a quick way to get some free nookie. Wiseman also comments about another Submissive friend who "has come to believe that there is a strong inverse relationship between how good a dominant a man is and how quickly he brings up the subject of fellatio." I'd laugh if I had not found this exact thing to be true.

Bullies & Manipulators
   Some people think that being a bully means they're being dominant. Bullies tell you how things are done and get upset when you disagree. Adults discuss the options respectfully. A real Dominant doesn't have to force you to do anything. Dominants who try to manipulate you into doing what they want are losers.

A Good Dominant May or May Not Be...

There are lots of things that people think makes someone a good Dominant, but in fact they really don't indicate much of anything. They include:

You Are Turned On

Just because someone makes you hot doesn't mean they know a darn thing about dominating. It could be pheromones or maybe they remind you of an old flame. It doesn't mean anything except that you are turned on.

Whether or Not They Initiate Contact

Some Dominants believe that initiating contact with Submissives is their nature and so they always take the lead. Others believe in allowing Submissives to be attracted to them. Neither is indicative of any innate ability to effectively dominate someone.

Their Ability To Write Well

Communication on the internet is predicated on being able to write and type well. Many intelligent people cannot do this, and many foolish people are unwilling to even run a spellcheck. I say foolish because writing riddled with wrongs makes a bad impression. This being said, being able to write well has nothing to do with being a good Dominant. It's still important to me personally because I'm a writer, but that's a different issue.

Privacy Issues

I never give out my real name or contact information to people I've only met online. And yet, I've found that Dominants, and particularly men who do the same thing get less respect. There are just as many unbalanced women online (Remember *Fatal Attraction*?) as there are unbalanced men. Don't give out your personal information, and also don't worry if they won't either.

What They Do For a Living

Yes, a stable person will have a stable job. But they don't need to be CEO of some corporation to be able to dominate. There is a stereotype of the female executive submitting in the bedroom, and the male househusband dominating, but neither are relevant. If ambition is important to you, fine. But it doesn't in itself indicate an ability to either dominate or submit.

Great Clothes

Anyone can buy fabulous leather outfits. Let them know you appreciate their clothing sense, then move on to more substantial topics.

Assertive Mannerisms

There's a huge difference between controlling situations, and controlling a person. Don't be fooled by people who act assertive in public.

Charm & Flirtatiousness

It might be fun to flirt with a charming Dominant, but social skills have little to do with the ability to control.

Paying for the Date

I used to think that the Dominant should pay for the date because they were the Dominant. On the other hand, some Dominants expect the Submissives to pay as an homage. A person may well be a fabulous Dominant, but is unemployed, low on cash, or may believe in equality outside the BDSM relationship. Several people I dated had met several Submissives before me, and were frankly tired of paying for all these dates that never went anywhere. The bottom line is that the person who asks for the date should pay for it. Don't play games like waiting for them to pick up the check - talk about it up front.

I've been getting to know Ronin, and it turns out that not only does he look like a fabulous Dominant, he also is one. But I didn't know this from his snakeskin boots, I learned it from how he responded to me over time. When it comes to judging domliness, only fools rush in.

Sadie Comes Out as a Bawdy Girl and so Much More

We tend to think of the erotic as an easy, tantalizing sexual arousal. I speak of the erotic as the deepest life force, a force which moves us toward living in a fundamental way.
~ Audre Lorde

The other day my sister asked me if I had ever known a man who was as sexually oriented as I was, not just in having or wanting sex, but in looking at the world through a sort of rose-colored sexual lens. After a few minutes thought, I realized that no, I hadn't. Sure, men love sex and spend a lot of time chasing it, but it's more than that. I look at the world from a paradigm of the erotic, which is expressed through my interests, my sense of humor, and the kind of people with whom I surround myself. My sister thought this mindset was something genetic in the women of our family since she and mom were the same way. She described me as a Mae West type, a bawdy girl. At last, an archetype which fits.

So, when I came out in the D/s community, such as it was, it wasn't a big dramatic moment. The moment arrived when I was chatting to my friend Zenobia, and I told her, with much hemming and hawing, about my sexual orientation. To my surprise she replied "Oh, I knew that!" It turns out she had a friend who was into the BDSM scene, and she had been tipped off by my everyday conversational language. As a writer, she was more attuned to those things, but it still surprised me that she could read me so easily.

Meeting My First Out Friend

Zenobia introduced me to her out and about friend Ethan. He was the first person I met who lived the BDSM scene in the open, with unfettered joy. I questioned him for hours as he explained how it all worked, and how he had suffered no ill effects from the process. While he talked, all I could think about was my own fears, of course. I was afraid if people knew, I'd lose credibility as a writer. I was afraid I wouldn't fit into the "leather" crowd, being a pretty typical Vermonter with an apartment, a job, an active church life, and so on. I was afraid, because I knew at the most intimate level, this would change my life.

Still, green as I was, I could see that BDSM folk experience a similar process of coming out that the lesbian/gay crowd has experienced for the last few decades. Both on a personal and a group level, we learn to accept our orientation, take the steps to pride, and the steps which release us from fear. The process for us is newer with so very few of us coming out of the BDSM closet. Only in this last decade are we blessed with the Internet and the monumental difference it makes in our access to information and our ability to build community, even in an obscure spot like Vermont.

I started my own coming out with research, reading, and exploring until I had an idea where I wanted to start. Then I had to come out to myself, which can be the hardest step of all. Issues of consentuality were always clear to me, and being brought up a Unitarian-Universalist, a religion with a liberal tradition, there was no residual guilt. So at least in the beginning, I felt very little conflict, but it sure did help having Ethan, who not only listened to me, but took me to my first munch. I am unusual I know. Many men struggle with their upbringing which taught them not to hit women, or that they were a wimp if they allowed someone to hit them. Women struggle with the specter of domestic violence which appears, on the surface, to have something to do with BDSM. For those of us who are feminists, we wonder how to reconcile a need to submit. Blessedly free from most of these issues, I jumped right into the dating scene.

Telling My Friends

My venue of choice for dating, there being no world wide web at the time, was alt.bondage.personals which was the first place I discovered information about BDSM, as well as a vast supply of dominant men, or at least men who said they were. As I learned how to talk to them about my own sexual orientation, I used these skills to also tell my friends about it, a process which became easier with each telling. Fortunately, my friends were mostly liberal intellectual types and the response varied from a vague disinterest to a smile accompanied by a raised eyebrow. I tailored my explanations to the sexual sophistication of the listener, being careful to make sure they didn't get caught up in silly stereotypes of Submissives being doormats or Dominants being abusers.

Most people have at one time or another engaged in a little silk-ties-to-the-bed type of bondage or a friendly spanking, so I used these common denominators to help them understand. I call it the "vanilla" version of D/s since these things are palatable to just about everyone. Sometimes I bring out a purple deerskin flogger so they can see how gentle and sexy the toy is. Not to mention the fact that it matches my outfits so well. Most importantly, I recognized that explaining D/s takes patience, so I gave each person sufficient time to absorb the information and ask questions. If they are ready and interested, we talk in more depth about things like the eroticism of pain and how serving can be a great gift.

A short word of warning here. Be sure to tell your friends that what you are telling them is absolutely confidential. This may be obvious to you, but this kind of juicy gossip can be a temptation. For example, one of my friends who didn't have strong boundaries "outed" me to another person. He didn't do it on purpose. He really just felt he was giving his friend additional information about me, but his way of explaining BDSM was unquestionably not the way I would have explained it. As a result, when I met this third party he treated me with less respect. Like it or not, based on the mores of our culture, it was natural for him to think I would hop in bed with him. I was never able to get this man over his initial impression of me, and so any possible friendship was doomed.

Joining A Community

The next step for many people is to join a D/s community like ours. But since I didn't have one to join, I started one. Of all the things I have done in my life, creating Rose & Thorn has been one of the most fulfilling. It has given people a safe place to explore their sexual selves. At the beginning, I had some fears about meeting people I knew, something which did in fact happen. At our second event someone from my church joined the group. After the initial awkwardness, we both realized we had an equal need for privacy, and I discovered my fears were unfounded. I have seen this same scenario play out with others who have encountered people they know with no ill effects to either party.

Where To Next?
   If I were to take the next step in my own "coming out," it would be to become an activist in the national BDSM community. For role models I have the many leaders who make up the BDSM Group Leaders association I belong to. They are an active force in educating the community at large, and we are all indebted to them and the other leading authors and activists who have given us legal support, safety in numbers, and information that was not easily available even ten short years ago.
   If you are considering sharing your "secret life" with someone, think carefully about whether this person is safe to open up to and how you will explain what you are doing. It helps to have some BDSM books on hand which will provide credibility. It can be enormously freeing to break the silence.

Pitfalls And Pratfalls
   For many people who have been raised under the conventional sexual mores of American culture, discovering their D/s orientation can let loose a torrent of needs. Having repressed their sexual desires for years, there is an urge to go wild and sleep and/or play with everyone who says yes. Although on the surface it can seem a great way to get experience fast, it is quite often the road to a broken heart, not to mention the risks of sexually transmitted diseases and inexperienced Dominants. D/s is powerful, and if you are new to the heady feeling of the power exchange, it can easily be mixed up with different powerful emotions like love, relationship, and commitment. If you decide to play actively, be aware that many of the new feelings you experience will not fit into your old frame of reference about relationships. For example, many people talk about very intimate details of their sex lives on a first date; intercourse is no longer an assumption of having a relationship with someone; and it is common for

people to enter a sexual relationship barely knowing each other.

On the other hand, I know several novices who read so much, and for so long, that they never actually experience anything. The thing is, you can read a hundred books and cruise a thousand websites and chatrooms, but it will not equal one hour of real experience. Education is very, very important, but is only as experiential as "describing" an orange. The live dynamic of interacting with someone is biting into an orange and feeling the juices run down your chin.

The worst pitfall of all is not to come out. When I was leader of Rose & Thorn, nearly every week someone contacted me inquiring about attending events, but who would be cheating on their partner/spouse. Of course we didn't allow them to attend because we believe in the "Consensual" of Safe, Sane and Consensual. Cheating on someone is clearly not consensual for the person being cheated on. Also, there was a very real risk of the hurt party discovering their partner's involvement in our group, then either crashing an event or violating the confidentiality of member's e-mail addresses. There's nothing like a scorned lover. We wanted guests to feel confident that everyone in our group was above board.

It is quite often these same people who have not yet come out to anyone. They live in ongoing fear of being exposed as well as the pressure of never being able to express their sexual orientation. Although it is undeniably scary to come out to a longtime partner, the alternative is so much worse. There are very serious risks to consider, especially if there are children involved, and those have to be weighed carefully. Still, I believe that repressing a primal force as powerful as one's sexuality can only, in the long run, hurt everyone.

So yes, I believe exploring that force is central to fulfillment in this life. You can chalk it up to my being a bawdy girl if you want, but if there is one thing I have heard over and over, it is that the gift of community provides safe passage for all of us.

Rough Sex, BDSM and other Mushy Deliniations

My first summer in Vermont I discovered Alberto selling collectible books at an outdoor flea market. Even as we flirted in the bright summer sunshine, he impulsively grabbed me and kissed me. I was astonished by a stranger kissing me, and took him as a lover that very weekend. Alberto was a lady's man, a man who loves women, who loves to please, and that pleased me.

I hung with Alberto because he liked rough sex, or at least he liked rough sex with me. I knew he did the slow hand thing with other women, but his dalliances didn't distract me any. He was the closest thing to BDSM when BDSM was just wishful thinking for me.

I have another lover now who is a lot like Alberto, although discovered under the aegis of the D/s community. Jeremy is one hell of a lay, and likes to please, too. More rough sex. Sometimes play rape scenes on the livingroom carpet. Sometimes the "39 steps" where I get a flick of tongue, a pat on the fanny, or a soulful kiss each time I took another step up. A lot of positions and a lot of hair pulling; a bit of rough and tumble as they used to say.

I like it well enough, although it doesn't seem much like BDSM to me. Jeremy thinks it is, though because he's a novice Dominant, and for the novice, moving from regular sex to regular sex with a spanking is BDSM. I don't argue with him. Let him have his delusions, as my mom used to say. They'll be forfeited soon enough.

Jeremy is also laboring under the misconception that after six months in the lifestyle, he has graduated from novice to intermediate. Maybe ten rolls in the hay with me plus some on the side. But does this a Dominant make? Perhaps, perhaps not. Depends on his state of mind I suppose. As I see it he was a great lay as a novice, and he's still a great lay as an "intermediate." But this still ain't BDSM.

I hope I'm not being too hard on him. I suppose some of my confusion stems from the night I first met him at a party. Just before we all went home, he knelt and laced up my party boots. His own submissive side is so close to the surface that I cannot easily see the Dominant he says he is. He's a switch, but to me his submissive side is what resonates. Maybe I'll always have that image of him in my mind, his soft grey eyes, bedroom eyes, gazing up at me.

His dominant style is not too different from his submissive style, pleasure oriented. He does whatever he can to make me happy, focussing wholly on giving me pleasure. The result is my feeling his submission to me, even though technically he's dominating me. He may be tossing me over the kitchen table to do me, but he's doing it because I want it. I'm not really sure what he would do if left to his own devices.

I wonder if there is a such a thing as "dominant" dominance and "submissive" dominance. In theory, if Jeremy wants to caress me all night long, it's my job as Submissive to go along with it. Not to mention it would be ludicrous to complain about too much. But somehow, something is missing and I'm not sure what that something is. There are touches of bondage, pain, control, but all hesitating, not followed through to someplace where I might forget myself. Never beyond lighthearted. There is more, but he's not there yet.

Rough sex can morph into BDSM, but where does one become the other? Fuzzy, very fuzzy. A novice or an intermediate? Depends on who's doing the measuring. A dominant Dominant or a submissive Dominant? Both or neither in the novice explorer. Is pleasure enough? No, not enough.

What is refreshing about Jeremy is that he is joyful and unfettered by "shoulds." He is a welcome change from some of the lifestyle folk who take BDSM so darn seriously. Together we gossip, we tickle, we giggle. Yes, we fuck. A lot.

Jeremy has no philosophy, no construct, no style. Not yet. Rather, he is present and rapt with passion. He kisses me impulsively, slides his hand into me, leaves me breathless. Maybe not BDSM, but enough to take him as my lover this weekend, and maybe longer.

Sobriquets and Screen Names: What we Call Ourselves

For a long time I called myself "Submissive Sadie." I liked the alliterative nature of the words, and I figured it was a fast way for people to know my BDSM orientation. I changed it to "Sensuous Sadie" when readers became confused by columns I'd written from a dominant point of view. Of course, even when I was "Submissive Sadie," lots of people didn't believe it anyway. These were usually novices; recognizable because they hadn't yet learned that you can't judge a book by its cover. Now that my name is neutral as to being Dominant or Submissive, there's less to be confused about. Or more. In any case, at least now I get less flak.

People often choose "scene" names when they join the larger community, figuring on hiding their identity as much as possible. There are legions of novices, and so we end up with a lot of scene names which sound just like any other name - Karen, Thomas, Susan, Bruce etc. Also common are names which have a submissive, sexual, or gender neutral quality such as Yielding, Candy, or Jamie. I chose "Sadie" for the combination of the unspoken "sexy" in Sadie as well as for the subconscious allusion to the

Marquis De Sade. For some reason, the name also reminds me of the Little Feat song "Sneakin' Sally Through the Alley" which isn't the same name, but expresses a mischievous and adventurous spirit.

Players also take on sobriquets ("An assumed name; a fanciful epithet or appellation; a nickname" according to dictionary.com) which express their orientation by use of an appellation. Examples are Madam Dragonfly, Domina Blue, Lady Midnite, and Mistress Tart. Some incorporate their interests into their names such as Master Stern, Lord Latex, or even Master Sparks. It's a bit harder for Submissives, who usually use tags such as Francis, boi of Mistress Juliana; Moby, property of Sadie; or barbie (Dex). There are a few which use the actual words of their orientation such as Submissive Steve or Slave Sandra but these seem to occur less often; maybe it's because they sound a little more awkward. Interestingly, there are also a number of pseudonyms which are relatively attribution neutral such as Sensuous Sadie, Queen Maureen, Binderup, and Ed the Czar.

There are also a number of courageous people who use their real and full names like Laura Goodwin, TammyJo Eckhart, Rick Umbaugh and Charlie Reid. Using their real names is in itself a statement of faith, that what we are doing is honorable, and they refuse to be ashamed. Laura explains: "I never had what is known as a scene name. I've always used my own name. That's because almost from the beginning I was public as a spokesperson for BDSM people. I never had a private, secret BDSM life. My BDSM life has always been public." Rick says, "The reason I am fully out is that it means I don't have to do the dance of the liar to cover for myself. Since I am a fully functioning, responsible human being with a great credit rating I have no reason to feel ashamed of anything I do, particularly in the privacy of my bedroom." Charlie adds, "I am who I am all the time and I'm not ashamed of anything I'm doing."

I am not this courageous. I've found that when vanilla people know this thing about your sexuality, they get distracted by this knowing, and it can become a barrier. I expect gays and lesbians get this feeling sometimes too, as if their sexuality had something to do with their work, families, or hobbies. It's just another sign of our culture's history of repressing that which is sexual in nature. Still, as my friend Leela says, "you can't exactly be in the closet if you're publishing your first BDSM book." She has a real point there, so I'm guessing at some point I'll be out of the closet entirely. All along I've been aware of the risks I've taken both as a leader and as a writer, so if that's what's in the cards for me, then so be it.

Some writers use full names which are completely fictional like Jack Rinella. Jack says, "My nom de plume came about because I was writing pornography and my real name is very uncommon. In fact all of us who have that last name in the US are closely related. So I fished around for another name."

I created a fictional name for the same reason as Jack. My real name is very unusual, and in fact is the only one in Vermont. My original thought was to use the full name Sadie Flatley; the Flatley after Michael Flatley the charismatic Irish dancer. Unfortunately few people recognized his name. Not to mention that Flatley does sound, well, a little bit flat. So Sensuous Sadie it is.

My friend Doug has quite the opposite approach. He feels the whole scene name phenom is silly, and he won't play. He's just plain Doug in vanilla life as well as in BDSM life. Sometimes it seems a little silly to me too, especially when someone who barely knows the first thing about being Dominant calls himself Master This or Lord That. A friend of mine told me about her Dominant who has her call him "My Lord." The problem is that it takes a lot of effort on her part to keep a straight face. He isn't anything she associates with a real Dominant, such as control, dependability, and power. She goes along for the fun of it anyway, a little role playing which works well as long as she keeps her real feelings about His Lordship in check.

In the traditional approach to BDSM these titles are earned, not taken on by choice. It's hard to imagine what "earning" a title would mean in a community which doesn't have a structure in place to manage these kinds of things. Some Dominants want everyone to refer to them as Master so-and-so, and I guess we pretty much have to go along. In any case, poseurs eventually unmask themselves. Jack Rinella's opinion is that "to assume a title like Master or Lord or even Sir is presumptuous and ought to be avoided. I don't tell people to call me anything except Jack. If they want to honor me with an honorific, that is their prerogative." Jack is more generous than I would be. I believe titles are earned, even for me. I don't want some strange Submissive calling me Mistress. As a turnabout on the old Submissive saying "I may be a sub, but I'm not your sub!" I say, "I may be a Dominant but I'm not your Dominant!"

A similar conundrum happens with capitalizing names. In the style of e.e. cummings, Submissives often do not capitalize their names in written communications. Examples such as karen or james, act as an effective visual aid to recognizing Submissives. On the emotional level it also seems to express in a visual way the sense of being submissive. I never use this style myself because for two reasons. It seems in some indefinable way to diminish the value of a Submissive. While we are Submissives and want to serve, there is sometimes a mistaken attitude that we are "less than" Dominants. Using lower case names or writing "Submissive" as "submissive" can encourage this kind of wrong thinking. The other reason is because I am a writer, and I follow standard rules of writing. Using things like lower case names, or the Instant Message style of writing such as "W/we" and "Y/you" take the reader away from the story, a cardinal no-no for writers.

    I may get less flak these days with my more neutral name, but people continue to struggle just as much with the idea that I am a switch and possibly a bisexual one at that. It's a bit mushy for our culture, which likes things black and white, clean and sharp, no ambiguities. So here's an option for you. Call me het sub Sadie if you wish, just don't expect me to call you back.

Making Sense of Internet Writing Styles

Some people write "We're going to the BDSM Ball," and some write "W/we're going to the BDSM Ball." Which is it really? This so-called "Internet-Style" of writing is a convention of chatrooms but has become prevalent in other places. The challenge is that when not in the chatroom, it can be confusing to readers who are unfamiliar with what it all means. Even worse, because it does not follow standard rules of English and is visually distracting, readers can become irritated and move on to something more agreeable. As a convention for chatrooms it is an useful mode of communication, but it may not be an effective communication style for other venues.

Internet writing style was born in the chatrooms, where a person is identified only by a typed name. It provides participants with an easy way to remember others in the room as well as identify gender and orientation, something particularly important when looking for a partner. One of the most common rules requires that Submissives uncapitalize their names, as in writing "sadie" instead of "Sadie." Others include using "W/we," instead of "we," or capitalizing pronouns such as "You" when referring to Dominants. Domme Harem writes that, "A sub should never capitalize themselves when saying i, me, my etc. and always cap the Domme when saying You, Your, She etc. This shows deference to the Dommes." Some might argue that deference and respect are earned, not granted simply because someone chooses to capitalize their name, but that's a different issue. Being a bit contrary myself, I might also wonder if capitalizing shows respect, does uncapitalizing proper nouns (names) reflect a lack of respect?

A similar set of rules has to do with entry into a chatroom. Sir Penguin writes that, "All Submissives/slaves are required to ask permission when entering or leaving the channel. It is considered respectful to do so. All Dom/mes are charged with the responsibility of granting this permission when requested." Despite Sir Penguin's pronouncements for his own website, rules are not at all consistent among chatrooms. Quite-Contrary-Mary discourages excessive formalities: "Upon entering the room, a simple 'hello' is fine. Please, no excessive greetings, walking around the room or anything similar. Remember there is a discussion in progress. Do not disturb it." In the first example, designating and respecting the status of the Dominants present is the focus, while in the second, readability and ease of use are more critical.

As do most specialized languages, Internet-Style differentiates the online BDSM community from the real time one. Lady Kat writes that "When Y/you are able to speak comfortably in this manner, Y/you will show O/others that Y/you have some experience and are serious about the lifestyle." Of course she is speaking to the online community as these conventions are not typical of the real time community, and obviously don't work when spoken aloud. But these rules do create a sense of bonding for the online community. Considering that many real time players do not take the cyber lifestyle very seriously, it is important that there be a safe space where that lifestyle is wholly valid. Group bonding is part of this validation, and an important way for online players to recognize each other both practically and figuratively. This is not unlike the BDSM community creating a safe space away from vanilla eyes.

For some Submissives, this style of writing has also developed as a sort of submission in itself. Shivante, a Submissive, comments that, "capitalizing any form of Master Thomas's name is an expression of endearment. Obviously i cannot bow my head, smile that smile, kneel, etc. for Him over the computer, so, i capitalize when i address Him or refer to Him."

Internet-Style writing can be an issue for the online players who prefer not to follow these rules. It can seem as if the rules were are pretty much handed down on Moses' tablet, and that people who don't follow them are not "real" Dominants or "real" Submissives. This, of course, is ridiculous. People who choose not to follow a particular protocol may do it because they consider themselves professional writers, simply don't want to bother, or because they feel that how you type is irrelevant to your BDSM lifestyle. Of course judgmental fools are hardly limited to the cyber lifestyle. The bottom line is that rules based on safety or privacy carry far more weight than arbitrary ones developed around how to type names and pronouns.

If this style of writing were kept strictly to the chatrooms, most people probably wouldn't care about it one way or another. The challenge is that many online players write this way all the time, whether or not it is appropriate to the venue. Many listservs ban this type of writing because it is difficult to read, and follows rules not widely known outside the online community. For example, I have observed that online players use the "W/we" designation quite often, but that still does not explain why they are doing that.

A related issue is that many of us capitalize "Dominant," but not "submissive." On the website DomSubNation.com, they explain that "The 'S' in sub was capitalized for a purpose, to be equal to the 'D' in dom. It is our belief that Dominants and Submissives are equal partners, in a relationship. We always felt uncomfortable in a lot of rooms where the 'D' towered over the 's,' looking down on it when we knew in fact the D/S we knew was nothing like that." In my own writing I capitalize "Dominant" when referring to a person, but not when it's an adjective such as in "she was acting dominant." To be consistent I realized that I should also be capitalizing "Submissive," and have done so ever since. There is no practical reason for not capitalizing Submissive, and all things being equal I recommend using consistent grammatical practices.

Writer Rebecca Brook agrees, commenting, "I happen to agree with you about the mutuality, but then, I'm a switch! I'm more comfortable with Submissives lower-casing themselves, though, than I am with Dominants lower-casing them. In other words, I like to make sure that the writing style is consensual!" This is an interesting point, as it's one thing to choose to type your name lower-case, and a whole other thing to have some Dominant do it for you. Using the non-gender specific "Dominant" is also far more effective than "Dom" or "Domme" unless you are specifically referring to a person. Aside from the obvious gaffs in pronunciation (they are pronounced the same), language should be as gender-free and sexism-free as possible.

Submissives often uncapitalize their name in what is known as the "e.e. cummings" style of writing (an author who wrote all in lower case). Some uncapitalize their name to identify the fact that they are Submissives, a convention which makes sense if it's important for people to know that fact. Unfortunately, in the English culture, lower-case words suggest that the reference is somehow diminutive, and this feeling of "less-than" is transferred to the Submissive by assimilation. I don't agree that Submissives are less than anything, so I don't ever uncapitalize my name. Of course, not all Dominants capitalize their names and not all Submissives don't capitalize theirs, so judging someone's orientation based in their typing is risky business. Some people even admit that they don't capitalize their own names not because of some deep meaning, but because they are lazy!

One Dominant I know insists on knowing the orientation of every person at an event because the way he interacts with people is based on whether or not they are Dominant, Submissive, or Switch. This probably works when he's at home around people he knows, but is quite ridiculous when anywhere else. I might even go so far as to say that treating anyone differently based solely on their orientation is disrespectful by its very nature. But then, that flies in the face of standard protocol, and we really don't want to go there. In real time events where formal protocol is not active, there is no clear way to identify your BDSM orientation. Even items like collars are often worn by both Dominants and Submissives. Not to mention that some collars are so jewelry-like that it would be hard to even know if they signified submission or just good taste in ornaments.

While it is critical to know a person's gender and orientation when you are looking to hit on them, this focus on knowing about someone's private life is invasive and downright nosy. We are not our genitals, who we sleep with, or whether we are the flogger or the floggee. What all these issues come down to is that the Dominant and the Submissive are equal players and should be written about with that in mind. Decima, founder of Fetish Fashion writes, "The relationship between Dominant and Submissive is essentially symbiotic in nature; it is mutually advantageous, one cannot exist without the other." Similarly, Columnist Rick Umbaugh writes that "We do not seek unity within individually (at least not the S/m part of our lives) but unity within our relationships. The yin and yang are separated into individuals, and individual roles and it is the practice of the scene, which creates the unity." In this model, the Submissive is an equal to the Dominant, not something less than in any way. If we truly believe that both Dominant and Submissive are integral to the BDSM interaction, then we should be respecting them equally in print.

One of the first things my editor taught me was that readers should be totally engaged with the story I'm telling, whether it be a quick e-mail to friends or the first chapter of a book. When you do something like write in non-standard English, which is what Internet-style writing is, you are taking the reader outside of the story. This cardinal sin is part of the reason why top-drawer publications like Prometheus do not publish articles in the Internet-Style.

Our writing style expresses a lot about us, quite often including things that we might rather not be communicating. For example, people who are too lazy to run a spellcheck tell us that they don't care about the message they're sending. You might say that you aren't a "writer" and so it does not matter how you communicate to others, but I would argue that if you want your audience to take you seriously, you may want to consider making your words free of spelling errors and in reasonably good grammar . While Internet-Style writing is not technically considered bad grammar, it is inappropriate for non chatroom situations if only because the majority of readers don't understand it.

The key difference is that when we write for our own pleasure we can write any way we wish. But when we are trying to get our ideas out to an audience, the medium is, indeed, the message.

References for this article

Spirituality In Slavehood
J. Mikael Togneri
http://www.leathernroses.com/submission/spiritualityslave.htm

Do Y/you really want M/me to type T/this?
Jonathan Krall
Prometheus, Issue #38

The Art of S/m
Rick Umbaugh
Nayat326@cs.com
This article can be found at Sadie's website at:
http://www.sensuoussadie.com/spiritualityarticles.htm

Virtual Time BDSM Safety
http://meltingpot.fortunecity.com/mali/18/vtbdsm.html

Lady Kat's BDSM Chat Rules & Guidelines
http://www.geocities.com/katrinatull/chatrules.html

Sir Penguin BDSM Chat Rules & Staff
http://www.sirpenguin.com/bdsm/chat/rules/

BDSM & Fetish Chat
http://qcmary.com/chat.html

Domme Harem Chat Guidelines
http://dommeharem.virtualave.net/guidelines/

Why I Don't Give a Hoot About Protocol and Why It's Important to Know Anyway

The first time I attempted to follow formal BDSM protocol it was a big fat failure. Part of the problem was that I was in a non-protocol setting. Not being able to identify whether a particular person was Dominant or Submissive put me in quite the quandary, not to mention trying to figure this out in the five seconds as they ran up and hugged me.

I was attempting this protocol feat because I was training with Master Dex of House Mermaid who appreciates the finer flavors of these kind of structured interactions. The truth is, I don't give a hoot about protocol. I'm not big on ceremony in general, and can be downright surly about rules in particular. I've even been told that I think the rules don't apply to me, which may well be true. I tend to see things like ceremony and regulations as artificial constructs, constructs which can assume more importance than the human connection.

I'm not saying rules are never important. Nor am I saying it's okay to disrespect fellow players. What I am saying is that following rules for their

own sake does nothing for my vanilla self and even less for my Submissive self.
 Let's back up a little bit here, because it's easy to get things mushed up. Information abounds on the rules of the BDSM game, and those rules vary a lot, just like recipes for spaghetti sauce. The general breakdown seems to be between etiquette and protocol. Etiquette is the good manners things we do at events which show respect for each other, such as not touching someone else's toys, respecting other people's kinks, and not outing people. I agree with this approach, not because of that hackneyed golden rule business, but because it's basic respect. Protocol tends to refer to the series of public interaction rules which grew out of our military history where the BDSM community was born. Master Dex describes the historical piece this way:

> "Much of the early protocols adopted in the lifestyle came from military servicepeople returning following World War II. Protocols between officers and enlisted personnel translated into the way Doms approached other Doms, Doms interacted with submissives, and subs interacted with other subs. These are general rules of conduct and behavior for when people and groups approach each other."

Common protocols you might hear about include things like Submissives not being allowed to sit on the furniture or avoiding eye contact with other Dominants. Dominants may be asked to "protect" other Submissives as well as not initiate contact directly with someone else's Submissive.
 Things sometimes get a little bit fuzzy, no matter how you differentiate between etiquette and protocol. At House Mermaid one of their protocols includes the statement "What goes on in the House stays in the House." Is this etiquette or protocol? Depends, I guess, on how you define it. Definitions aside it's a good rule which shows

respect for what happens in the house. Lord Battista of the Erotic Power Exchange Dominion elaborates: "All facets of our life have protocols. There is the way we treat each other, the simple protocol of welcoming a new person to our neighborhood, the way we greet an old friend with a handshake, or for us bikers a hardy hug and a pat on the back."

It is the protocol part of things which leaves me cold. For people who dig the ceremony, the structure, the clear rules, protocol can be a reflection of their inner self. Some others, the artistic temperamental types, prefer to wriggle our own way. I often feel quite silly when attempting to follow formal protocol, and feeling silly doesn't add anything to my Submissive experience. I don't see that it makes a jot of difference where I'm sitting or whether or not I put my hand out first to shake someone's hand.

The handkerchief code is an example of a construct in our community, not part of protocol per se, but similar in its history and structure. The hanky code helps people identify each other's orientation, the left jean's pocket for Dominants and the right pocket for Submissives. Since I don't wear jeans to scene events, or in fact anywhere, I don't have anyplace to put a colored hanky. Not to mention, as my friend Gary Switch points out, that there's no middle pocket for us switches. In the subdued lighting of most events I've attended, I'd have to peer pretty close at someone's ass to figure out whether the darn thing was light pink (dildo fucker) or dark pink (tit torturer). Mixing these up could be a mistake of serious proportions. You might be willing to argue this code is or is not defined as protocol, which is one thing, but as an example of a set of rules, I find it impractical and confusing.

It is in things like the hanky code where people can mistake the form of BDSM for the content of BDSM. Form is the toys, the fashion, the community, and, the protocol. These are the accoutrements of our lifestyle, physical manifestations which represent what we're feeling, not the experience of Dom or Subspace itself. It's certainly true that I love scene fashion as much as the next girl, and also true that I never wear heels higher than 1.5 inches. Do I think fabulous 6" heels are cool? Sure I do. But they are not what being Dominant or Submissive is about.

So this is my take on the protocol thing. Sure it's a bit loosey goosey, but then so am I. Given this you might be surprised to know that the other night I stood up and gave a mildly impassioned speech about why we should all know and care about protocol. I received a few raised eyebrows of course, being my feelings about this particular topic are well known.

I think of formal protocol as Emily Post for the BDSM world, manners to smooth the way between different ways of living, of which we have many. Holding your fork like a shovel and scooping food into your open maw may work fine at home, but won't fly at a dinner party. Wearing jeans might be great at a munch, but wear them to an office with a dress code and you sure will lose your chance at a promotion. In this context, there are plenty of good reasons to know some kind of basic rules. Knowing the protocol of your group or community gains you entre and respect because you cared enough to be aware of the community standards.

Depending on the flavor of your community, protocol may or may not be practiced actively. Even if you aren't using it much at home, eventually you'll travel a bit and want to be easily accepted into other communities. The key thing is to check out the groups before leaving and so do the "when in Rome" thing when you get there.

Lastly, formal protocol is an important part of the BDSM community's history. Why is history important? Well, it may not be for you personally, but our community would not be here without the many people who have fought to get us here. Groups like the National Coalition for Sexual Freedom are still fighting for us today, both in the legal and the political arenas. I've been reading lately about people who have been prosecuted for private BDSM practices and groups who have had events cancelled because of closed-minded religious freaks. Even with this, we have the freedom to congregate and explore our lifestyles mostly freely. Many of us have the choice to come out and know that our legal rights will be protected. Thank our foremothers and forefathers for providing us this mature community. Thanking them means knowing a little bit about how our community developed.

At that first party where I tried to follow formal protocol, I didn't do such a great job. But at least I'll know that I made the choice to know what the rules were, even if my performance was a big fat failure. What counts to Master Dex and to me was the effort.

Part VI
Becoming "Sensuous Sadie"

The most interesting thing about being a scene personality is that my personae, Sensuous Sadie, has become a bit detached from the real me; the actual person who tap-tap-taps away at her computer in her jammies; a grilled velveeta sandwich at hand. Sensuous Sadie is a very real part of me, but she's also a vital and spiritual force of her own. Learning to be in the spotlight, with all the glamour and weirdness that entails, has been quite an experience. I've been on the soapbox for many of my ideas, some of which have driven a few of my readers a bit batty. I invite you to read about my experiences in becoming a leader and a writer.

SCENEprofiles Interview with Sensuous Sadie

SensuousSadie@aol.com
www.sensuoussadie.com

This is a compilations of questions asked of me over the years. "Cal" stands for Community at Large.

Cal: In January of 2002 you were quietly going about your business, running Rose & Thorn and writing a few friendly columns on the side. Now your writing is being published in several magazines and more. What's this about?

Sadie: "The funny thing is that it all started when my job was cut to part time in March of 2002. This was the same week that I officially became the first Leader Emeritus of Rose & Thorn, a combination which resulted in a fair bit of grief as well as a significant increase in free time. At first I was a little disoriented, but then I realized I had this incredible opportunity. First I learned how to design websites, and soon had designed my own as well as several others. It helped a lot that I have a graphic design background, which is reflected in the original graphics on my website.

"During this time, I discovered that I have a facility for doing interviews. I enjoy researching what other authors have written and asking them questions about it. Naturally, I started with BDSM group leaders, but now that I've moved away from leadership I'm concentrating on well-known authors because they have a broader appeal to a national audience. I am fascinated by their perspective on the scene as well as their complex ideas about their own BDSM practice. My hope is to collect these interviews into a compilation.

"All this writing had to go somewhere, so in addition to running them in my own newsletter *SCENEsubmissions*, I started sending them out to other magazines, both paper and online. I currently have columns and interviews running in a growing number of publications including the *BDSM News, Prometheus, Leatherpage* and many more. There's an updated list of these publications on my website. It took a lot of organization because of course each publication deserves a certain number of pieces that haven't been published before; I didn't want any of my columns or interviews to get overexposed. Fortunately, my experience in writing gave me a good idea for what editors were looking for.

"I look back on the last year or so and I can see a radical difference both in my personal writing life as well as in my personae as Sensuous Sadie. It's very satisfying because I receive a lot of e-mail from readers who really enjoy my columns and interviews. They comment that my style is very validating of all kinds of BDSM expression. You could say that being cut back on my job turned out to be a huge blessing in disguise."

Cal: I read a quote about you that I'd like you to respond to. Yielding, a columnist (http://www.bdsmu.com/) said, "Sadie is

possibly the most vibrant and informed individual on the internet today. She never sleeps due to a surgically implanted device that allows her to labor tirelessly on her newsletter, her website, her very fascinating interviews, her BDSM writers Yahoo group, her leadership of Rose & Thorn, and very likely 30 or 40 more BDSM related activities I haven't yet run across. I respect her for her strong opinions, and for being able to convey them without diminishing the validity of other ideas." I can't help but wonder why you do all this stuff, and what keeps you motivated?

Sadie: "The most common misconception I've found is that people think I'm making tons of money off all these projects. In fact, I have yet to make one cent from any of it. Hopefully the book will sell and at least pay for the cost of self publishing it. Obviously, it's not about money for me.

For a long time I was a writer in the vanilla spirituality market, which was great - but I don't think I ever reached more than the 20,000 readers who read that particular publication. Now I still write about spirituality, but with a BDSM twist. Unlike the spirituality market which is well saturated, there are many opportunities (unpaid ones) on the internet to publish my writing. As a result, you could say that I found my niche here. There is a large audience hungry for information, particularly for information about the "soft" side of BDSM - the emotions, spirituality, and relationship side of things. There are tons of "how-to" pieces out there, but few that deal with the actual experience of being a Submissive or Dominant.

I do have a mission, which until now I've never really articulated. Over the last few years I came to appreciate the power of community and how it validates our lifestyle. I feel that frank discussion about BDSM is the only way to help both kinky folk and the larger community understand that what we are doing is a healthy and creative approach to sexuality. It's not for everyone, but for those of us who want to pursue it, we deserve to be able to do so without fear.

Cal: Another quote. This one from Chris M, writer and Emeritus Board Member of Black Rose (http://subbondage.net/chris_m/), who also drew your snake BDSM logo: "Sensuous Sadie's website not only offers the best collection of writings on the web examining the intersection of the spirit and sadoerotic, but it is also simply one of the most illuminating collections of SM writings period. Think of it as a continuation of the essays of Mark Thompson's *Leatherfolk* **tailored to the cyber age and the new millennium. Simply Wonderful!" That's pretty high praise. The intersection of BDSM and spirituality seems to be the focus you've moved into bigtime. What's that about?**

Sadie: "That is one heck of a compliment from Chris, especially since I have read *Leatherfolk* as part of the research I've been doing. It's a wonderful book. As I mentioned, I have been interested in exploring spirituality for a long time. I'm also working on my second book which is about BDSM and spirituality, and you can read my introduction to this on my website www.sensuoussadie.com. As part of my research for this I've been reading the many articles on the subject, and wanted to create a place where people interested in the subject could find everything in one place. The result is this large section on my website with many guest authors, including Chris M.'s excellent work.

"I am also planning on collecting these writings into my second book. There are a few books that look at BDSM and spirituality from a female Dominant or gay perspective, but none dealing with this amazingly complex and intricate subject in a broad way for heterosexuals. The themes that resonate for me have to do with using pain as a conduit to spiritual expression, ideas that are well represented in the work and writings of authors Fakir Musafar and Cleo Dubois."

Cal: What's the deal with the book? Why publish your columns?

Sadie: "Fundamentally, writing is what writers do, and so I want my message to be heard. There are plenty of books out there on how to tie someone up or whatever. My book is more about the emotional journey. I suppose a little bit of it is vanity as well. It's pretty exciting to think of your writing out there in published form. I'm hoping to reach a national audience."

Cal: Your newsletter *SCENEsubmissions* now focuses on BDSM and spirituality. How did that come about?

Sadie: "The newsletter started out as a venue for Rose & Thorn to make announcements. Over time, I started including columns, poetry and other information and it grew to a very informative weekly event. When I stepped down from Rose & Thorn, we decided to detach it from Rose & Thorn because it had really become "Sadie's Newsletter" and also it had become national in scope.

"There are plenty of books about BDSM, but for the most part, people aren't charging down to the bookstore to buy those books. Maybe it's because they are embarrassed or maybe they just don't feel committed enough to the lifestyle to buy a book on it. It's easy and anonymous for these folks to get my e-mail newsletter. There's no commitment or cost involved. I see this as the perfect opportunity to get these people the information they need, even if they don't know they need it yet.

"I have a very strong belief in accessibility. If information is hard to find, or difficult to read, it won't achieve its purpose of communicating. The newsletter provides quality information in a friendly and accessible format. As I was collecting those great articles on BDSM and spirituality that I mentioned already, I started running them in the newsletter and got very positive feedback because at the moment, there are no other publications with this focus. On a personal note I've really enjoyed the contacts I've made with scene people; we are a wonderful and diverse group."

Cal: The photos on your website project a glamorous image. Is that real?

Sadie: "When I think of 'glamour,' I imagine women in sleek leather outfits knocking around the New York City nightlife. It's hard to think of myself as glamorous or sophisticated because I live a fairly quiet life, not to mention the fact that I'm living that fairly quiet life in Vermont. I do think of myself as a sophisticated thinker, and that is probably reflected in my writing. I have a background in marketing, so I have a very good idea of how important it is for readers to think I'm glamorous, and that's why my photos look the way they do. Selling my image helps me sell my writing."

Cal: How did you become aware of your BDSM orientation?

Sadie: "I discovered my sexuality and even my submissiveness fairly early, but of course didn't have a name for it way back in high school. What

I did know was that I wanted my boyfriend to be more assertive with me sexually. He was submissive himself, a pattern I discovered in my boyfriends a few years ago. I know I have a powerful personae, and it naturally attracts submissive men. I remember making bets with boyfriends where the loser would have to be 'slave' for the night. Of course I lost the bets on purpose, but even so they rarely were able to be as dominant as I wanted. This has been a real problem for me, and I've had to consciously choose different kinds of partners."

Cal: For the record, are you Dominant or Submissive? Straight, bi or lesbian?

Sadie: "Technically, I am a switch. However, as my experience evolved I discovered I have difficulty maintaining a relationship where I am Dominant. Maybe I'm just lazy, but it seems like too much darn work. I'm guessing an attitude like that delineates this is not my natural inclination. Nowadays, I consider myself eighty-five percent Submissive, and fifteen percent Dominant. In other words, I prefer to submit, but darned if occasionally I don't get the urge to bend some guy over my maple table and spank the hooey out of him.

"Part of the reason dominance is work for me is because I'm a highly analytical person, very goal oriented. I tend to plan out my scenes in great detail and do something exciting and creative each and every time. I enjoy planning a lot, but even so, this approach is difficult to maintain in a long-term relationship. A big part of what I get out of my own submission is the joy of release, of letting go and turning it over. I make decisions all day; I don't want to be making them in the bedroom.

"I consider myself heterosexual. Men's bodies have a visceral effect on me, and that is the foundation of my sexuality. Also, I'm something of a Don Juan. I see the beauty and sexual quality of every man, or most of them anyway. This gift doesn't mean I sleep around though, only that I can really see the special gift of every person I meet. I have also had a number of experiences with women, both in vanilla relationships and one in BDSM, mostly when I was in my early 20's. I enjoy looking at women's bodies and flirting with them, but I don't usually take the next step into a relationship. I'm open to the possibility however. I have an attraction to butchy dominant type women. "

Cal: Why did you change your name from Submissive Sadie to Sensuous Sadie?

Sadie: "I called myself Submissive Sadie for many years. I liked the name because it advertised my orientation as well as had a nice sound. Unfortunately I often wrote from the perspective of a Dominant, which became confusing to my readers. I decided to change my name to express not my specific orientation, but my general approach to life. I particularly like the name Sensuous Sadie because it's alliterative in multiple ways."

Cal: There is an ongoing debate about whether the BDSM orientation is genetically based, or something we choose. What's your take on this?

Sadie: "My friend Mal brought this up one evening over dinner. He was seeing a psychologist who was convinced that the BDSM orientation was a choice, a bad choice. The shrink was trying to convince Mal he should go 'straight' if you will, and try to have relationships with non-BDSM oriented women. My feeling is this: it doesn't matter a wit how your orientation came to be or how you express it. What counts is that we feel fulfilled and happy in the expression of our natures. If Mal didn't like how he felt when exploring BDSM, then it's a good thing for him to find out what it's about and create a new way of living. But for me, I love expressing my sexuality this way. It feels whole and real to me. That's the bottom line; if it feels good then it's okay. I don't mean 'good' in the superficial hedonistic sense, but good on a spiritual level."

Cal: You also edit the Reading Room at the Erotic Power Exchange Dominion. What is your interest in this?

Sadie: "I met Lord Battista who is the Webmaster of EPE Dominion when I was looking for a BDSM-friendly host for the Rose & Thorn website. There are only a few kink-friendly website hosts, and Lord Battista spent a lot of time helping me get up to speed on my newly learned website skills. I manage the reading room there, and it's been a great place to archive a lot of material which was first published in the newsletter. Since I don't publish fiction in the newsletter, it also turned out to be a great venue for stories, humor and other items. It's a nice balance. I also have enjoyed getting to know Lord Battista who is a remarkably grounded human being, as well as dedicated to supporting the BDSM community in a variety of ways."

Cal: There's been a few incidents on New England Listservs where you were flamed for your ideas as well as some of the interviews you did. Why do you think this happened?

Sadie: "That's a very interesting question. I have given some thought to it, and even have a little theory of my own. I am a female leader who is outspoken, as well as a writer who has a platform in my columns and the various places they are published. To make things more complicated, I am submissive, something which seems to bug a fair number of Dominants, mostly men. Some feel a Submissive can't be in charge of something as successful as Rose & Thorn, which of course I think is ridiculous. A fair number of people have problems with the female leader thing too, although most of the BDSM groups I'm aware of have female leaders.

"Being a writer has something to do with it, too. I'm a good writer and I know it. Whenever you put your ideas out there, it's an invitation for all the people who disagree with you to get their panties in a twist. I'm considerate toward readers who respectfully disagree with me, but I pay no mind to people who use profanity and are irrational. I think it bugs them I don't bite, if you know what I mean.

"This approach has definitely rubbed a number of people the wrong way, which is too bad. I guess they feel a leader should be accessible to them in all ways, and not have boundaries. Others think I should never make mistakes. I do make them, and when I do they're on display bigtime. One of my weaknesses is that I really have a problem with irrational people, and I avoid them. This sometimes causes problems, but I haven't really found a better way to deal with it.

"Sometimes I think some parts of BDSM are a construct in certain ways, with rules of conduct and so on. I also think of life as a construct in that each of us creates the way we will see the world. There are objects like an apple or a computer which pretty much have the same reality for everyone in the sense that they are indisputable by definition. What is interesting is how people respond and react to those objects. To me, my computer is a tool to go about my daily life. To another person it's something to be feared. Same object, different response.

"This same difference in response happened when I made decisions for Rose & Thorn. People would do hurtful and obnoxious things, but I soon realized their actions have to do with their own fears, and are not about me. I have learned to not take things personally, not just on the superficial level but in really believing and understanding that their reactions are about their own perspective. As a result I can usually respond in a rational way, even as I detach from the emotions swirling around. My life construct helps me understand that people come from their own experiences in their reactions to me.

"The bottom line is that I have very strong boundaries, and I know who I am. I have high expectations about my communications with people in that they be respectful and rational."

Cal: Why did you start Rose & Thorn of Vermont?

Sadie: "In June of 1999 I had been with my partner Ryan for about two and a half years. Ryan was what I call a 'cheerful Dominant' for his lighthearted and joyful approach to dominance. He's an artsy type with a sexy streak of femininity. When he decided to move south I was pretty bummed because I wasn't really in the mood to start dating again. Frankly it took me a while to find Ryan, and dating Dominants can be arduous. A lot of them aren't really dominant; they're just plain pushy.

"One morning as I was sunbathing, I came up with the idea to create a BDSM group. I'd been to a few munches and things like that, but the groups always disappeared after a few months. It wasn't for lack of interest, but because the leaders weren't very organized. Running a BDSM group is not about BDSM, but about running a business. I figured it would be a snap because I know a lot about business, and I'm very organized. I had this list of people who'd contacted me over the years I'd been single, so I sent out an e-mail and got the ball rolling. So I suppose you could really say it was enlightened self-interest to start with. It was later on that I developed a sense of the group as something which was bigger than just me, something about building a community.

"People often thank me for having started Rose & Thorn because it freed them to explore their orientation. My response is that I didn't really do it for them, I did it for me. That's not me being ingenuous either. In a way, everything you have to do has to be for yourself. It's not that people don't appreciate what I do, but I faced a fair bit of criticism when I was in the leadership role. People often thought that Rose & Thorn policy was my personal policy as if I was persecuting them personally. So all along I've tried to keep in my mind that I'm acting out of my own best interest. My sense of self is connected to my spiritual self, so when I say I did it for me, it was in the more global sense. I believe we are all connected on a soul level."

Cal: How did your leadership inform your BDSM practice?

Sadie: "Getting involved in the community did change my personal practice of D/s. Before Rose & Thorn, I dated a lot of Dominants I met on the Internet. I gained a good bit of experience from dating so many men, who varied from complete novices to experienced players. I only got involved with a few of them, but having so much choice helped me recognize my value in the scene both as a woman and a Submissive. I had many more choices than most men in the scene, and this awareness meant I didn't have to accept the first Dominant who happened along.

"Part of what gets Submissives into trouble, especially in the beginning, is that they're so desperate to experience BDSM, they get involved with just about anyone who rings their bell. A dangerous proposition.

"The best part about being involved in a community is the sense of the big picture. Having met literally hundreds of Dominants, I have a very good idea of what's real and what's not. I've also become much more careful about who I play with. In the beginning, I would sometimes play with a Dominant just because he turned me on. I soon discovered that just like in vanilla relationships, lust alone is insufficient to maintain a relationship.

"Unfortunately, a lot of people are attracted to the BDSM lifestyle because of its dramatic side: the role playing, the power exchange, the clothing. I've met many Dominants, particularly male ones, who use BDSM as a sort of cover for their inability to connect on an emotional level. In the beginning, I was fooled by Dominants who were good looking, had charisma, dressed well, and had a 'Dominant' personae. I soon realized these things are easy to fashion. Real Dominance is a deep and visceral thing, something, which has nothing to do with the trappings of BDSM. Being able to recognize these differences has been the most useful skill I've developed.

"One of the challenges I've found is that the mantle of leadership can be intimidating to potential partners. Part of it is that anyone who shows up as my date at local events is bound to get a lot of attention. This worked out pretty well for the two Submissives I've had in the last few years. However, I get the feeling that for the

Dominants I've dated, the public thing is a bit harder. After all, when I'm in leadership mode, I'm a bit dominant myself which can cause a problem with competitiveness. I expect some of it has to do with the fact that it took me nearly three years to attend a public event with a Dominant for the first time, and so it naturally attracted a fair bit of attention. It's a very strange thing, but I'm well aware that people gossip about me, presumably because of my leadership role. That puts a lot of unfair pressure on any Dominant with whom I get involved, something along the lines of 'Gee, who is this guy who can actually dominate Sadie?' The reality of my submission is that I love to give it up, but it's hard for outsiders to see because of my outgoing personality."

Cal: Why did you step down from your leadership role with Rose & Thorn?

Sadie: "The funny thing about leadership is that people assume there must have been strife of some kind. It's really quite unfortunate, but understandable when you hear about some of the dramatic coups happening in the leadership boards of other BDSM groups. I'm proud, and admittedly relieved, that Rose & Thorn's core group is an integrated and cohesive group.

"In interviewing other leaders I discovered there are two schools of thought on leadership of BDSM groups. Many of the leaders believe in the dictatorship approach or 'benevolent dictator' as I always thought of myself. Others believe it's important for there to be a board where responsibility and change is voted on by many, including sometimes the community involved. The difficult part of this approach is that egos and power politics are common and can destroy a group. I feel the one leader approach is more effective, but maybe that's only because it's the way I did it. I do believe that once a group grows to a certain size, a board is needed to manage the complexities of a larger organization. I found running the actual group to be pretty easy. I'm very organized and had it down to a system which functioned efficiently.

"What I wasn't getting from leadership was connections with smaller groups of people who were of a like mind. I take a spiritual and emotional approach to BDSM, and I wanted to spend more time with people who took that same approach. I also felt that if I was not in a leadership position, I might be able to express my submissive side a little more in public. It's quite impossible to be even remotely submissive when you are in charge of a complex organization. Now that I'm free to do what I want, I can explore this part of myself a little more."

Cal: How has your life changed since you are no longer leading Rose & Thorn?

Sadie: "The biggest difference is that the drama quotient has gone from about ninety-five percent to five percent, something which I very much appreciate. When you are a leader, you have to reply diplomatically to everyone whether or not you like or respect them. As a writer, I only have to please myself. If someone, or a particular publication doesn't like what I write, I simply move on to another publication.

"I've also discovered that coming out to friends is easier. In the past I not only had to explain not only BDSM but the idea that there were groups, and that I was leading one. Nowadays I just say that I am a sex columnist, something which people are already familiar with through the writings of authors like Susie Bright. In other words, I now identify primarily as a sex columnist rather than a group leader.

"Interestingly, I was so focused on work for a while there that I spent nearly a year being celibate. It's a little amusing really that I was writing about sex and relationships but not having any. I do believe that there are periods in life when you focus on one thing or another - work or relationships or family. This was my work period. I could have had a lover if I wanted one, but other things were more important."

Cal: What are your hopes for the future of the Vermont community?

Sadie: "My main interest is in seeing Rose & Thorn and the other local groups grow and prosper, which they are clearly doing. We have an extremely competent management team now in charge, and I feel confident they will continue to do a great job.

"I've been quite thrilled that the Vermont Society of Kink started up here about a year ago. Having another group takes a lot of pressure off of Rose & Thorn to be all things to all people. I'm hoping the community continues to grow, and that eventually we have a number of groups all working together. I know that can be a challenge, because I see the strife happening in some other states. Still, I'm hoping we can avoid those situations, and we've certainly done a good job so far.

"Even though I don't generally participate in play parties, I'd like to see more of them happening locally. I think they are a great venue for people to learn from each other. It's a challenge since Vermont has such a small community and we have a limited number of experienced players, many of whom don't have the facilities or the interest in hosting play parties.

"I've always been focused on making connections between our community and the larger BDSM community of New England. I hope we continue to nurture those relationships, because it's the connections with the broader community which create a safe atmosphere to explore our own orientation."

Arrogant, Hysterical, and Nearly Insane: Being a BDSM Writer

Yesterday, my friend Carson commented that writing helped me communicate with myself, release tension, and remain sane. He hit the mark on the first two counts, but my sanity has never been at risk. I am a pretty stable person, both mentally and corporally, although I did find his vision of me entertaining.

Reading my writing makes people feel they know me and in a way they do, but in another way they don't. I recently read some e-mail feedback accusing me of being arrogant and hysterical. There's a lot of things people could accuse me of which have merit; perhaps that I am too "type A" or act like an ice queen, the opposite of a drama queen. But arrogant or hysterical? Those words reflect the reader's fears, not me. With examples like this, it's easy to isolate fact from interpretation. Unfortunately, there is no way to identify the Truth, with a capital T, of anything. I doubt such a thing even exists in this universe with so many ideas of what's right, and such a vast unknown. This concept of relativism is also expressed in the story of Rashoman where an event happens and is described by a series of witnesses. Same event, same "truth," but completely different interpretations.

In the writing world, readers have their own Rashoman experience as they interpret what they read. Once my writing passes into their brain, it takes on a different cast, one tinted by their fears, passions, and personality. That's why they sometimes come back at me with words like arrogant and hysterical. My words have passed into another realm, the realm of their inner life, and through the journey are altered beyond recognition.

Novelist Tim O'Brien refers to two different kinds of truth. There is "happening truth," the indisputable reality of what happened, and "story truth," the personal colorized version of what happened. The things I write about did happen, but often not in the order or exact way I described them, also known as poetic license. Even so, there is no "indisputable truth" of my experiences. I have even entertained the idea there are no real "facts," not even the kind which seem indisputable like owning a cat or the sun shining. This discussion hasn't been resolved yet, and probably will never be. In a way, I'm telling the "story truth" here, because it's the only truth there is, my truth for me. The only thing which is True, with a capital T, is that my writing comes from a spiritual source, so while the details might not be true in an absolute sense, they are true on a more fundamental level.

Knowing what I write is often misunderstood or misinterpreted, you might wonder why bother? I write because writing drives me. It is a spiritual expression, and has been part of my healing process in the last two years, coinciding with my recovery from my last relationship. I was always a writer of one sort or another, but writing in this genre has changed my practice as I increasingly focused not on the mechanics, but on the "erotica mystica" of D/s .

There are a lot of BDSM books out there, books which describe those practicals of the lifestyle. How-to this, How-to that. I thought of the big name writers as being glamorous and I wondered where I fit into this hierarchy of activists, group leaders, and highly trained specialists. It's one thing to scribble musings and post them on my website, but another to look a famous person in the eye and know we're both on the same path. I am no expert in BDSM, no specialist in anything particular except following my heart. Would this be enough?

In comparing myself in this way, I made a mistake, a big one. I bought into the pecking order so common in our community. Perhaps it's because of our historically military underpinnings, but this doesn't explain it all either. I think a lot of it has to do with the fact that the foundation of the D/s experience is about power, and the exchange of power. Because our community attracts more people who enjoy this aspect, it's natural for power struggles to occur on a group and community level. While politicking is also common in vanilla groups, I have found that in my own life the vanilla part, work, social life, and so forth, are pretty much drama free. It is the BDSM community where I have observed so many issues approached from a substructure of fear and competition.

Unfortunately, these hierarchies are not based on intrinsic human value, but on an artificial construct. Some put a premium on being an expert, a group leader, or an activist. Some value people by how many play parties they've been to, whether or not they are partnered up and for how long, or which group they affiliate with. Sometimes it's "eye candy" appeal with the best trophy-Submissive or trophy-Dominant winning.

I have been evaluated by these standards, sometimes succeeding and sometimes failing to measure up, depending on who's doing the measuring. I'll even admit I've sometimes valued one scene person over another because of these artificial standards. Now I see my error. My validity comes from speaking my own truth, from acting from the heart. I am a spelunker with a writing muse, exploring the caves of the power exchange with one hand clutching my Nancy Drew flashlight and the other tap-tapping my keyboard. There is no validity to succeed or fail at; I just am and that is enough.

    I also take a non-traditional approach to sharing my ideas. I believe the universe is abundant, and by allowing my ideas to be heard freely, I express my faith. Fellow writers worry no one will buy my book if much of it is on the website. They fear my ideas will be stolen, and I will lose out big time. They don't understand that my ideas can't be stolen. Wherever they go, and however they are used is exactly how they are meant to be used. By sharing my work, I perpetuate abundance and share my faith. By speaking out for acceptance and inclusion, I validate myself and connect with my spiritual self. By refusing to be afraid, I give courage to those who are.

    Some may say these ideas are arrogant, hysterical, and possibly one step from insane, but I say it's just the writer's muse.

Top Three Reasons Why Readers Think I'm Full-o-Hooey

If you're doing it, it's real.
- Dossie Easton and Catherine A. Liszt

I received an e-mail last weekend from a local reader "Brian," who hates my columns and decided and it was darn tootin' time to tell me that I had "no experience to speak of in the BDSM world." He felt that only long-time leather men and women, long-time as in twenty, thirty or forty years in the scene, had the right to write about their experiences.

How long have I been in the scene? Good question. If we're talking about the Vermont scene, you could say I've been knee deep since the "early" days, which would be 1999 when I founded the first BDSM group here. Brian's right on that score; a leatherwoman I'm not. Perhaps instead you could measure by when I first had a long-term D/s relationship, which would put me about ten years in the "scene" even though there was no scene to speak of round these parts. Or, if you wanted, you could count my first formal BDSM experience which was in college, some twenty years ago.

Considering that I can't figure out how to calculate my official years, I wonder how Brian performed his calculations. In any case, I don't believe that time, in itself, is an indicator of anything. My friend Dex of House Mermaid has been involved with BDSM for only about four years now. During this time he has been fully engaged in a 24/7 relationship, making his four years about equal to forty years of dabbling. Not to mention that Dex is totally committed to the BDSM lifestyle. Not only does he practice the single tail nearly every day, he does this on top of writing a leather column and hosting monthly play parties and workshops.

It also bothers me that Brian thinks I don't have the "right" to write about my experiences. Does he imagine that there is some certification for BDSM writers? In contrast, I believe that no one has to justify their right to self expression. Of course there is a skill issue involved when it comes to writing professionally, but I doubt even Brian would say that my wordsmithing isn't good enough for the dozen magazines that publish my work.

I wouldn't mind so much if he just told me that he thought my ideas were stupid and that was the end of it. He has the right to his opinion after all. But how can I take a person seriously who says I shouldn't be writing because I'm not a real "leatherwoman?" Heck, despite my Harley jacket left over from my riding days, no one is every likely to classify me as a leather anything. At nearly forty, I'm a lot of things, but a tough leather babe isn't one of them.

Brian is not the only person to tell me that my ideas, experiences, and writing are invalid for reasons not connected to those actual ideas, experiences, and writing. The same week of Brian's silly whining, I received an e-mail from "Toni," who couldn't stand the fact that I write both from a Dominant and Submissive standpoint. Writing from both perspectives makes sense to me, since I'm a Switch, and in fact I sometimes even do it even in the same column as you will read below. I do this because it's important for people to see that Dominance and Submission are like yin and yang in that they are not opposite ends of the continuum, but different expressions of the same power exchange. Toni wanted me to take some kind of stand although she clearly didn't believe me anyway, stating, "I do not believe you have either a Dominant or submissive sexuality, but, rather, like many in the scene, only a sensualist looking for some sort of high or some kind of attention." I considered having my Dominant Griffin write her an e-mail confirming my actual state of submission, but instead told her that I wouldn't be at all offended if she didn't read my writing.

The final nail in my coffin of zero credibility is the fact that I rarely play in public. As most readers know from my series on the subject, play parties just aren't my thing. I prefer to do intimate things in a private intimate space, finding that my most powerful experiences occur when I not distracted by the theatrics that public play entails.

Although play parties are supposed to be confidential, there are always stories floating about afterward about who did what to whom, and at what degree of style and sophistication they did it. One of the casualties of these stories was my friend Elizabeth who could really hold a room with her mystical style. A while back she was roundly attacked by a few protocol nazis who did not approve of the particular safe words she was using, and who made false accusations that she was an "unsafe player." Sadly, she no longer feels safe in expressing this beautiful part of herself in public. What a great loss to all of us.

Knowing that I would be in the spotlight as she was, I can't help but feel even less motivated to attend public play events. What if I were, for example, to make a mistake? Last weekend when

213

dominating Griffin, one of my flogger tails accidentally hit his balls. I apologized immediately and gave him a hug, but these things do happen, I can just imagine the fracas if this had happened in public; reputations have been destroyed for less.

I suppose you could say that this is my manifesto for what lies at the heart of credibility. I want to be judged on the excellence of my ideas, not on the length of my stay at the BDSM hotel. I want readers to laugh or weep at my stories, not at how I label my orientation. I want to sink or swim on my own merits, not on whether or not Griffin spanked my ass at some silly play party last weekend.

In the bigger picture, this kind of critical approach to one another reflects the larger problems of our community where the politics of our community makes for cranky bedpartners. Perhaps this happens because so many of us are control freaks, or because as a sexual minority we still react from a place of fear. Whatever the reason, every time a fanatic like Toni tells me that my way of doing BDSM is not good enough, not real enough, it's one more kick in the ass of cohesiveness in our community. If Toni cannot accept that I do BDSM differently than her, how will we ever convince our vanilla brethren that what we're doing is okay?

If I sound a bit on my high horse, well I probably am - born of suffering fools ungladly. All I ask is this: don't waste my time with silly admonitions about how you think I should or should not live my life. If you don't like my ideas, or think I'm wrong, then tell me your opinions and I might change my mind. Allow me to take a different approach to BDSM than you do. Support a diversity of opinion. Add your voice to the mix, even if you aren't a professional writer. By accepting differences on the personal level, we create a world where eventually our differences will be accepted by the vanilla community and beyond. Whether or not I am a "real" leatherwoman is irrelevant. What counts is the level of integrity I lived in my own life, and shared with others. I encourage you to do the same.

Controversial... Me?

Any good writing is mildly controversial.
~ Lord Battista

    Last week someone told me my writing was considered mildly controversial. My fur ruffled a bit over that. Hell, I write about spiritual things. I write about my experiences in the BDSM world. I write about openness and inclusion and finding your own path. How could such blandness be controversial?
    But then I got to thinking about some of the comments I'd received.
    In my column about deciding whether or not to attend play parties, one reader felt I didn't have sufficient experience to write about the subject. Do I have enough experience? Maybe not by her standards, but definitely by mine. In any case, my writing should stand on its own. If what I write makes sense, then the exact number of times I've been to play parties is irrelevant.
    In my column about coming out, I wrote that each of us must be honest about our sexuality with ourselves and our loved ones. One reader protested that I wasn't considering the consequences of coming out. He was right. I'm not considering those consequences because I don't know what they are; each person has a different

situation. I'm still going to say it and write it; I believe it.

In my series of columns on how the BDSM scene in Vermont is inclusive, some readers complained that I didn't have a right to speak for all of us. I agree, and I encourage them to write about their views. Still, it's not like I was advocating anything illegal, immoral or dangerous.

Maybe, as Lord Battista says, it's not so much the content of my writing, but that I have a platform. Yes, I have a personae, Sensuous Sadie. Yes, I have a newsletter and a website. Yes, I'm a good writer, and I have something to say. Most people don't have any of these things. A fellow writer told me that these facts are, in themselves, enough to foment insurrection.

I wonder if the very fact that I am writing is an irritant to some readers? I know it's a special gift. When I write, it's like my higher power is speaking through me, something magical. On the other hand, I'm not stopping anybody else from writing up a storm, for my newsletter or anyone else's. And I do run all letters to the editor, whether or not the readers think I'm full of hooey.

My friend Leela tells me that anytime you write about your beliefs, it's controversial by definition. Anytime you speak out, all the people who disagree with you will consider your views "controversial." However, she reminds me that if my intentions are from the heart, readers will know that. If my intention were to be controversial, people will be right to slam me for it too.

I wonder what controversial really means. When I write, I speak from my own truth, about what I believe is right for me. I write about freedom to choose in a culture which is often delineated on rules of one sort of another. Many players feel it's important to follow the party line, to practice BDSM their way. I argue for freedom to follow your own path, as long as you play safe, sane, and consensual.

Maybe this is heretical. Maybe it's just too risky to encourage people to think independently. Maybe in a world where religion and work and sexuality are packaged up nice and neat, someone suggesting we be present and accounted for shakes things up.

At the end of all this is just me and what I have to say. For the readers who are moved by what I say, thank you. That's why I write, to allow my heart to speak to yours. It's not courage which keeps me putting it out there, but that I'm a writer, and that's what we do. Otherwise, it's just filler... controversial filler.

Appendix

There are a lot of specialized terms in the BDSM scene, some of which I've included here. This list is not comprehensive, so if you want to read more I encourage you to visit the website below which has more information on the lifestyle. I chose this particular glossary because the author, subaltern, has a sense of humor about what we do which comes out in her writing. It's important to explain our lifestyle in a way that people can understand what we are doing, but it's also important not to take the whole thing too seriously.
~ Sadie

Glossary of BDSM Terms

By subaltern

Reprinted with permission from Malcolm Lawrence, Editor in Chief of Babel –The multilingual, multicultural online journal and community of arts and ideas.
http://www.towerofbabel.com

More terms can be found at:
http://www.towerofbabel.com/sections/erotica/submittedforyourapproval/indexofterminology/

BDSM: It stands for Bondage & Discipline, Dominance & Submission, Sadism & Masochism.

BONDAGE: The practice of restraining your victim. This most commonly involves rope, but can also involve chains, leather straps.

DISCIPLINE: Discipline can have various meanings. It can be a synonym for a system of training. It can also be what happens to you when you are bad. Play discipline (or play punishment) is a term that denotes that a punishment is not serious, but strictly for fun.

DOMINANCE: Dominance basically means that one has been given some measure of control by the submissive person (this level obviously varies) and in exchange for the submissive's obedience, the dominant takes control and assumes the responsibility of caring for the submissive and for both partners' general well-being, either for the purpose of a scene or for a longer period of time.

DOMINANT: also Dom (male), Domme (female): A Dominant is one who derives emotional and/or erotic satisfaction from a partner's surrender of control. This could be surrender of control in erotic situations only, or in varying levels of life decision-making, or both. A dominant is often also (but not necessarily) a sadist.

S&M: (Sadism & Masochism, or SM, S/M): Used to denote the physical activity of pain given and received.

SADIST: One who receives erotic pleasure from the application of pain. A sadist is NOT: a wife-beater, a rapist, a serial killer, a kicker of dogs and a stealer of candy from babies. This misconception is common. While it is certainly not impossible that an erotic sadist could be any or all of these things, it is not common and by no means true across the board. Your average erotic sadist is interested in mutual gratification with a consenting partner, and in using all kinds of pain as pleasure-giving stimuli. Forget those whip-wielding weirdoes you saw on Springer the other day; they aren't exactly representative.

MASOCHIST: A masochist is a person who receives pleasure from receiving the sadist's ministrations. A masochist is NOT: a person who has a massive orgasm every time they stub their toe (what I think of as the flipside to the "sadist as dogkicker" stereotype); a person who gets off on root canals; a person who enjoys being poked and prodded and fondled by random strangers in bars; a person who owns a video copy of "John Tesh Live At Red Rocks," or a person who loves tax time.

SCENE: Roughly analogous to Leatherfolk or Leather Community, and when used in this way it is usually preceded by "the," as in the Scene. It refers to any or all aggregates/groups of people who do what it is that "we do." the Scene can refer generally to all people involved in "WIITWD," or it can refer to all the people involved in "WIITWD" in a particular geographic area (e.g., New York scene) or with a particular sexual orientation (e.g., Gay scene). In this sense it is also frequently used as a qualifier, e.g., Scene Folk, Scene People.

SUBMISSION: See submissive below. Submission involves the gift of some level of power/control by the submissive to the dominant, and the gift of obedience. In return, the submissive will be cared and provided for, and (hopefully) lavished with attention and sensation, either during a Scene or for a longer period of time.

SUBSPACE: This can mean one of two things. Which one will usually be apparent from context.
1. The vast majority of submissives are not in a submissive frame of mind all the time, but only under certain circumstances, at certain times and situations. Like the Dominant, the submissive must also make a deliberate effort to access this part of his or her consciousness. This is also often referred to as being in a submissive headspace.

2. Subspace has another meaning which is considerably more difficult to define, especially for those who have never been there. The best way I know how to describe it is that it is like a spiritually transcendent state of complete and overwhelming bliss, the aftereffects of which can last for hours and even days. I have heard it

referred to as "a spiritual high." While this is happening, the submissive/bottom is often said to be flying. It is similar to, but exponentially more intense and powerful than, what is often called "runner's high."

Lecture Mode On: An understandable mistake that many, many vanillas make is thinking that all of this fancy stuff we do is solely for the purpose of a physical orgasm, that this is really just very weird and baroque foreplay. I'm not knocking orgasms; I like 'em as much as the next girl, but subspace and Domspace are often really what we're ultimately trying to achieve. Many of us, myself and He Who Must Be Obeyed most definitely included, are also quite fond of vanilla sex as well, and yes, I like kissing and caressing and oral lovemaking, and come when someone stimulates my clitoris, just like the average vanilla woman does. Lecture Mode: Off.

SUBMISSIVE (also sub, or *yuck* subbie): A submissive is one who derives emotional and/or erotic satisfaction from surrendering some level of control to a dominant. A submissive is often also (but not necessarily) a masochist.

POWER EXCHANGE: The commonly used term for play that involves some exchange of control or power. This can occur over the course of a scene or for a longer period of time.

SAFEWORD: A code word that stops the scene cold. Used when someone has had all they can take. Some use a system of red (stop), yellow (slow down, lessen the intensity), and green (go ahead, dammit, I love it!). Others just have one word. When the submissive/bottom is gagged or for other reasons cannot speak, some specified signal, e.g., dropping a handkerchief, can serve as a safeword.

SCENE: The second meaning of the word, usually used with a verb as in "to do a scene" or as a verb, e.g., sceneing (also playing). This refers to performing some or all of the activities referred to above. A scene can be as complex or as simple as the participants deem it. It can be whacking your partner a few times with a hairbrush and then ordering them to satisfy you orally, or it can involve elaborate bondage, 500 clothespins, chains, whipped cream, knives, and large scarecrows named Sven.

SSC: An acronym for "Safe, Sane, Consensual." There is naturally much disagreement as to how the individual terms safe, sane, and consensual should be defined, since obviously some level of risk is always going to be present. In some circles this term has a negative connotation, standing in as a codeword for a "gentrified" overly: safe brand of "WIITWD. In others it is completely neutral; how it is being used can be easily determined by context.

SWITCH:
A switch is:
Someone who can be both a masochist and a sadist.
Someone who can be both a submissive and a Dominant.

A switch is NOT:
Someone who can't make up his or her mind what to be. Someone who of necessity cannot be serious about dominance/submission or sadism/masochism, because of said "flightiness."

I think the best way to understand it is to think of a switch as the perverted equivalent of a bisexual. These relationships are no shallower just because they are capable of being both Dominant and submissive.

VANILLA: A person who doesn't do "WIITWD." In some circles this is derogatory, but usually it is a neutral term. It is used both as a noun e.g., "My ex-wife was a vanilla" and an adjective e.g., "We had vanilla sex yesterday."

WIITWD: an acronym that stands for "what it is that we do." It is in very common use as being a rather non-specific term; it can be used without implying any sort of value judgments or narrow-mindedness concerning specific types of kink.

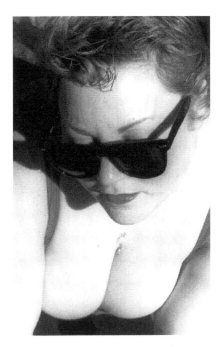

About the Author

Sensuous Sadie is a BDSM columnist and edits *SCENEsubmissions*, an online newsletter. She founded Rose & Thorn, Vermont's first BDSM group in 1999 and led the group until March of 2002 when she passed on the leadership to the current director. She now devotes her time to writing, both for her columns and her series of interviews with scene personalities called *SCENEprofiles*.

Sadie lives in northern Vermont and has a great passion for its beautiful Green Mountains. She is an avid portrait photographer, works out religiously and spoils her cat Spencer, who she describes as "not remotely submissive."

Sadie can be reached at:

SensuousSadie@aol.com
www.sensuoussadie.com

Why I self-published this book

Some time ago a publisher expressed interest in collecting my columns into a book, and we worked on the project for a year. At the end of this year, I realized that for a variety of reasons, this process was just not working for me. I decided instead to self publish with Trafford publishing, who has been as responsive and responsible as any writer could wish. I particularly appreciate the fact that by self-publishing I could design my own cover and layout and make it exactly the way I wanted to (yes, I'm a bit of a control freak). There is also no editor standing over my shoulder telling me what to write or not to write about. I would recommend Trafford to any writer who wants to get published. You can find information on them at www.trafford.com.

ISBN 1412001830-8

Made in the USA
San Bernardino, CA
13 March 2013